# HANDBOOK OF FETAL HEART RATE MONITORING

D1570193

# HANDBOOK OF FETAL HEART RATE MONITORING

Second Edition

## Julian T. Parer, M.D., Ph.D.

Professor of Obstetrics,
Department of Obstetrics, Gynecology and Reproductive Sciences,
Associate Staff, Cardiovascular Research Institute,
University of California, San Francisco, California

**W.B. SAUNDERS COMPANY**

A Division of Harcourt Brace & Company
Philadelphia London Toronto Montreal Sydney Tokyo

**W.B. SAUNDERS COMPANY**
*A Division of Harcourt Brace & Company*

The Curtis Center
Independence Square West
Philadelphia, Pennsylvania 19106

**Library of Congress Cataloging-in-Publication Data**

Parer, J. T.
    Handbook of fetal heart rate monitoring / Julian T. Parer.—2nd
ed.
        p.    cm.
    Includes bibliographical references and index.
    ISBN 0-7216-3639-X
    1. Fetal heart rate monitoring.      I. Title.
    [DNLM: 1. Fetal Heart—physiology.    2. Fetal Monitoring—methods.
    3. Heart Rate—physiology.      WQ 209 P228h 1997]
    RG628.3.H42P37    1997
    618.3'20754—dc21
    DNLM/DLC
                                                        96-37238

HANDBOOK OF FETAL HEART RATE MONITORING        ISBN-0-7216-3639-X

Printed in the United States of America.

Last digit is the print number:   9   8   7   6   5   4   3   2   1

*For Pip*

# ■ *Acknowledgments*

Any system of clinical management evolves over a period of time, and is subjected to much modification and refinement. The best environment for such refinement is in pragmatic and critical usage, and this I have been fortunate to find at the University of California at San Francisco. There is little reticence regarding the challenging of ideas at this university, and for this I am grateful to my fellow Faculty, Midwives, Fellows, Residents, Medical Students, Nurses, Nursing Students, and many others involved in the care of pregnant mothers and their unborn children. It is through such critical input that the management approaches described in this book have emerged.

I would like to thank Ms. Christine Thatcher for her careful manuscript preparation, Ms. Kathy Safford for help over the years with aspects of antepartum testing, and Ms. Phoebe Grigg for her help with art work.

# ■ *Preface to the First Edition, 1983*

In less than two decades, fetal heart rate monitoring has achieved broad acceptance as a valuable aid in optimizing fetal outcome in the United States and elsewhere. This acceptance has not occurred without vigorous controversy, and in many spheres of monitoring, the controversy continues. However, a consensus is being reached about the role of monitoring and interpretation of fetal heart rate patterns.

Initially, interpretations were made by empirical observations of human beings, relating heart rate pattern to outcome. Theories regarding the patterns were developed on the basis of little experimentation because such studies rarely are possible in human beings, particularly treatments resulting in asphyxia. The more recent advances—and those which are likely to be the most dramatic in terms of improving the accuracy of interpretation—are being made after deliberate manipulation of animal fetuses. It is only through such experimental studies that the mechanisms of fetal heart rate changes, fetal asphyxic compensations and protective mechanisms can be determined.

There is little doubt that the third decade of monitoring will see a great increase in such knowledge. However, I believe that fetal heart rate monitoring will remain the basic screening technique for the clinical determination of the adequacy of fetal oxygenation. The major change is likely to involve an improvement in interpretation and in learning to distinguish fetuses that are merely "stressed" from those that have impending cardiorespiratory decompensation (i.e., "distressed" fetuses).

This book is the result of many years of involvement in fetal physiology and fetal heart rate monitoring. I give great credit and profound thanks to the numerous mentors who have guided and assisted me through research and training at various institutions. Among them are: Emeritus Professor N.T.M. Yeates (University of New England, New South Wales, Australia); Dr. James Metcalfe (University of Oregon Medical School, Portland); Dr. Kent Ueland (formerly of University of Washington School of Medicine, Seattle); and Drs. E.J. Quilligan, E. Hon, C.B. Martin, Jr., W.J. Ledger, Roger Freeman, Richard Paul and B.S. Schifrin (while at Los Angeles County/University of Southern California Medical Center, Los Angeles).

I acknowledge with gratitude the atmosphere for scholarly progress provided by the Cardiovascular Research Institute and the Department of Obstetrics, Gynecology and Reproductive Sciences at the University of California, San Francisco and the Nuffield Institute for Medical Research and the John Radcliffe Hospital, University of Oxford, where I spent a year of sabbatical leave. My colleagues and collaborators have provided a stimulating testing ground and hearty cynicism for many of the basic and clinical theories outlined here.

J.T. PARER

# ■ *Preface*

When the *Handbook of Fetal Heart Rate Monitoring* was published in the early 1980s, the general definitions and principles had been laid down and the techniques had been in relatively widespread use for about a decade.

Since then a huge literature on the subject has developed, and publications contain numerous recommendations for use of fetal heart rate (FHR) monitoring in limiting fetal asphyxial morbidity. Fetal heart rate monitors are found in virtually all North American delivery rooms, and the majority of babies have at least some electronic monitoring. However, enthusiasm for the technique is no longer universal, because in the dozen or so controlled trials that have appeared from around the world little benefit could be shown, and there appeared to be increased Cesarean section rates in the monitored mothers. This dampened enthusiasm has been of benefit, because it has caused a serious examination of why FHR monitoring is not living up to its early promise in actual clinical usage. Here are three examples of recent optimistic advances.

1. The most recent metaanalysis of the randomized controlled trials shows that newborn seizures are halved with electronic monitoring compared with auscultation. Cesarean section rates are, however, increased 20% (see Chapter 15).

2. A serious effort is being made in North America to standardize FHR pattern interpretation in an objective, unambiguous way, so that all investigators and clinicians can use the same definitions (Chapter 9). This is of particular importance as we appear to be on the threshold of computerized FHR analysis.

3. Intelligent computer systems for improving interpretation and teaching of FHR monitoring, and decreasing intervention, are being developed. Such studies suggest that expertise can be achieved in FHR interpretation, but that in the hands of the untrained and inexperienced, electronic FHR monitoring offers little benefit over auscultation (Chapter 15).

These are exciting times for the technique of electronic FHR monitoring, and improvement in its application can be expected this decade. This manual places particular emphasis on the physiologic basis of FHR pattern etiology, and hence the biologic plausibility of the technique. The manual describes a management system which has been refined over two decades, and has worked well in clinical practice in San Francisco.

J.T. Parer, M.D., Ph.D.
San Francisco, 1996

# ■ *Contents*

# ■ *Part One*

ANTEPARTUM

# ■ *Chapter One*

# The Evolution of Fetal Surveillance

 EVOLUTION OF TECHNIQUES FOR FETAL ASSESSMENT

Twenty years ago fetal health in the antepartum and intrapartum period was being assessed by a combination of clinical tests, largely nonspecific, which clinicians generally regarded as bearing some relation to fetal outcome, and a scattering of newer, purportedly more specific tests relating to some objective measurement of the fetus. The clinical evaluations included categorization as "high" or "low" risk pregnancy, estimates of fetal size or fundal height, passage of meconium, irregularity of auscultated fetal heart rate, and subjective evaluation of fetal movement. The more objective evaluations, just gaining a degree of clinical use in the early 1970s, included continuous fetal heart rate monitoring; static ultrasound imaging (B-scans); hormonal tests, such as estriol and human chorionic somatomammotropin (HCS) levels; and tests of pulmonary maturity in amniotic fluid, such as the lecithin:sphingomyelin (L:S) ratio, creatinine concentration; and the "shake" or "foam" test.

There has been a remarkable refinement and enlargement (or extension) of many of these tests in the last two decades, primarily due to the development of reasonably priced, high-resolution, real-time ultrasound, and of an understanding of the relationship between aspects of fetal behavior or state and fetal health.

Although "intervention" and early delivery had been practiced for decades in certain pregnancies (e.g., Rh alloimmunization, maternal diabetes mellitus), the combination of a number of tests of fetal condition, and of pulmonary maturity, has allowed the important concept of optimal timing of delivery in complicated pregnancies. This process allows the obstetric team to make decisions regarding the continued risk of remaining in utero versus the potential risk of sequelae of prematurity.

## II DETERMINATION OF FETAL GROWTH

Clinical estimates of fetal weight and progression of fundal height measurements still have a place in management today, particularly as screening tools. The hormonal measurements (estriol and HCS) have all but disappeared from North American obstetrics.

The standard technique for ultimately determining fetal size today is to obtain sonographically determined fetal measurements: head diameter and circumference, abdominal circumference, and femur length. These are weighted by a formula and a fetal weight is automatically calculated in most modern ultrasound imaging machines. The percentile based on either known menstrual dates or sonographically determined dates is also given. Both the estimated fetal weight (EFW) and centiles are of value in confirming whether a fetus is small or large for gestational age. Serial measurements can be used to detect the appropriateness or otherwise of fetal growth. The EFW has a standard deviation of about 10 percent, relatively similar to that of clinically estimated fetal weight. Most machines will give the gestational age equivalents for each of the above four measurements, allowing the clinician to look for internal consistency and also to note head/abdomen discordance, which is usually seen with later gestational intrauterine growth restriction.

## III DOPPLER VELOCIMETRY

Many ultrasound machines are equipped with a device for measuring Doppler velocimetry in the fetal vessels, particularly the umbilical artery and middle cerebral artery. This device gives an index of vascular impedance in downstream beds, and in the umbilical artery increased systolic:diastolic indices are related to decreased fetal placental blood flow. In the middle cerebral artery the resistance may decrease as the fetus compensates for nutrient or oxygen limitations, so indicating increased cerebral blood flow.

There are many strong advocates of the use of Doppler velocimetry in clinical management, and abnormal tests have been related to increased stillbirth and other morbid outcomes. The role of Doppler velocimetry in clinical management utilizing other biophysical tests is still being established.

## DETERMINATION OF ADEQUACY OF FETAL OXYGENATION

Soon after the introduction of continuous fetal heart rate monitoring for intrapartum assessment, the technique began to be used for antepartum assessment also. The most popular test in North America was the contraction stress test (CST, or oxytocin challenge test), whereas a small group of Europeans concentrated on the presence of fetal heart rate variability in the monitor tracings, and thus forshadowed the nonstress test (NST) by a decade or more. These tests served well for the 70s but many voiced concerns over the high false-positive (i.e., falsely abnormal) rates, up to 80 percent for the NST and 50 percent for the CST. The biophysical profile (BPP) was therefore a welcome introduction, with a false-positive rate less than the previous tests. The accuracy of this test is enhanced by a combination of factors: fetal movement, fetal flexion tone, fetal breathing, amniotic fluid volume, and the NST.

There has now evolved a hierarchy of tests of fetal assessment, of increasing complexity and decreasing false-positive rates. The series consists of (a) fetal movement counting (kick counts), (b) the NST, and (c) the BPP, or modified BPP. On certain occasions the CST may be used as a follow-up to an abnormal or suspicious NST, or it may be used subsequent to an equivocal BPP.

 ## DISEASE SPECIFIC TESTING

Of great importance is the relatively recent realization that antepartum testing needs to be disease specific. For example, the volume of amniotic fluid can decrease over a period of days in the postdate pregnancy, so evaluation needs to be done at least twice weekly for this indication. In the case of fetal anemia due to Rh isoimmunization, the BPP may be 8/10 even with a fetal hematocrit below 20 percent, but the NST will be abnormally smoothed and lack accelerations, and one can usually provoke late decelerations with contractions. Again, in fulminant preeclampsia weekly NST testing may not be adequate to detect fetal deterioration when there is a rapid decrease in placental function.

 ## APPROPRIATE INTERVENTION AND TIMING OF DELIVERY

The above tests for determining adequacy of fetal growth, and fetal oxygenation, have allowed many babies to be delivered before death or damage in utero has occurred. However, such successes would not have been possible without a number of other parallel developments: (a) detection of fetal developmental defects by genetic testing and ultrasound imaging; (b) tertiary referral centers; (c) neonatal intensive care units; (d) tests of fetal pulmonary maturity such as the L:S ratio, phosphotidylglycerol, and rapid surfactant tests; (e) glucocorticoid treatment for accelerating fetal pulmonary maturity (primarily betamethasone); and more recently, (f) neonatal surfactant administration.

We are almost certainly not at the end of the evolutionary trail in the development and application of these technologies. There is no doubt, however, that our ability to determine the condition of the fetus, and more accurately detect its state of health, and our ability to rationally intervene and optimally time delivery, has vastly improved in recent decades.

The most important challenges for the future are to refine these techniques to prevent overintervention due to the prevalence of false-positive (i.e., falsely abnormal) results in many of the tests, and to ensure a proper understanding of these tests by the providers of obstetric health care.

The purpose of this manual is to examine one of these techniques, fetal heart rate monitoring, and to present a simple system of interpretation and management based on physiologic principles and empiric observations, which will largely avoid false negatives and minimize false positives.

# ■ *Chapter Two*

# Antepartum Fetal Heart Rate Testing

The clinical methods available for detecting impending or actual fetal asphyxia are limited to quantitation of fetal movement, electronic beat-to-beat fetal heart rate (FHR) measurement, the biophysical profile, and transvaginal fetal blood sampling. Only the first three can be used clinically before rupture of membranes or with a closed cervix. The other tests of fetal surveillance, such as high-risk classification and ultrasound imaging, help us only to decide which fetuses require more definitive testing. These tests are relatively poor predictors of intrauterine asphyxia. Cordocentesis for fetal blood acid-base and blood gas determinations has been used in an investigative setting, but is not of practical use in a clinical setting. Doppler velocimetry of fetal vessels has strong advocates, but its role in combination with other techniques of fetal surveillance has yet to reach consensus.

An approach to antepartum surveillance includes the following:

- Basic screening with fetal movement counting.[8, 15, 17]
- Nonstress testing (NST) in cases of suspicious kick counts or in certain high-risk situations.[4, 11]
- Biophysical profile (BPP)[13] or contraction stress testing (CST)[7] in the presence of nonreactive or suspicious NST.
- In the case of a suspicious or positive CST, the BPP may be done in an infant so premature that delivery seems unwarranted. Similarly, in the case of a low value on BPP, the CST may be used as backup test, and if normal, delivery may be able to be delayed in cases of extreme prematurity.

There is continued controversy regarding the relative merits and efficacy[22] of these approaches, although they are now well established in clinical practice.

# NONSTRESS TESTING, INCLUDING VIBROACOUSTIC STIMULATION

Nonstress testing (NST) consists of detecting the FHR, fetal movement, and uterine activity by external means, and noting long-term variability and accelerations of FHR with fetal movement. These parameters have been shown to be predictive of fetal outcome.

## A Technique

Twenty minutes of a good-quality FHR and tokodynamometer tracing are obtained with the patient in the semi-Fowler's position or with a left lateral tilt. Blood pressure measurements may be taken at intervals. Fetal movements may be signified by maternal sensation, attendant's observation or palpation of the maternal abdomen, and sharp upward marks on the tokodynamometer tracing. Some recently introduced FHR monitors are able to simultaneously detect fetal movement with an inbuilt Doppler system.

Fetuses have been observed to have inactive sleep cycles that often last 20 to 40 minutes, and may last up to twice this time. These periods, assumed to represent non-REM (rapid eye movement) sleep, are usually associated with reduced FHR variability[18] (Fig. 2–1). If the fetus is initially inactive, it may be stimulated by vibroacoustic stimulation (VAS) or manual stimulation, or the mother may be given appropriate liquid to ensure an adequate glucose level. However, the utility of these latter two maneuvers has been questioned.

The operator or mother marks on the record any fetal movement and notes whether the FHR accelerates to at least 15 beats/min above the baseline, with a duration of 15 seconds above the baseline with the movement. The baseline FHR is "normal" if it is within the range of 110 to 160 beats/min. The long-term amplitude variability (i.e., the irregular crude oscillations of 3 to 6 cycles/min) should have an amplitude of 6 beats/min or more on the external monitor. The beat-to-beat or short-term variability cannot always reliably be read with the Doppler ultrasound device.

Vibroacoustic stimulation depends on the fetal response to an acoustic stimulation (generally produced by an artificial larynx) applied to the maternal abdomen over the vertex. This test has been validated and shortens the time required to produce a reactive test.[21] The usual approach is to give a 1-second stimulation in the nonreactive fetus, and repeat after 1 minute if there is no acceleration response. A second repeat may be done with 2 seconds of VAS. Sometimes small variable decelerations occur after stimulation; they are not considered to be pathologic.

## STATE CRITERIA

| State criteria | State 1F | State 2F | State 3F | State 4F |
|---|---|---|---|---|
| Body movements | Incidental | Periodic | Absent | Continuous |
| Eye movements | Absent | Present | Present | Present |
| Heart rate pattern | A | B | C | D |

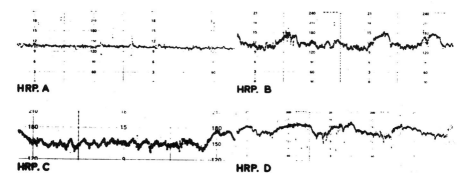

**FIGURE 2–1.**    The relationship between fetal state and typical FHR patterns. F1 corresponds to non-REM sleep, F2 to REM sleep, F3 to quiet wakefulness, and F4 to active wakefulness. Note the reduced, but not absent, FHR variability in F1, the normal FHR variability in F2, and almost constant accelerations in F4, giving a tachycardia as the accelerations become confluent. (From van Vliet MAT, Martin CB Jr, Nijhuis JG, Prechtl HFR. The relationship between fetal activity and behavioral states and fetal breathing movements in normal and growth-retarded fetuses. Am J Obstet Gynecol 1985; 153:582–588. Used by permission.)

## B Interpretation

The following set of criteria for interpretation is one of several used successfully in various institutions.[11, 20]

1. Reactive fetus: At least two fetal movements in 20 minutes with acceleration of FHR reaching a peak of at least 15 beats/min and lasting 15 seconds; long-term variability amplitude of at least 6 beats/min; baseline rate within normal range (Figs. 2–2, 2–3). Reactivity may be either spontaneous or provoked by stimulation.

2. Nonreactive fetus: No fetal movements or no acceleration of heart rate with movements or stimulation; generally poor or no long-term variability; baseline rate may be within or outside the normal range (Fig. 2–4).

*Text continued on page 13*

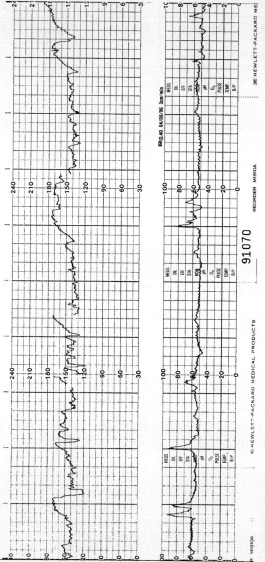

**FIGURE 2–2.** A reactive fetus, showing marked accelerations of more than 30 beats/min with fetal movements. The spikes on the tokodynamometer channel indicate the movements.

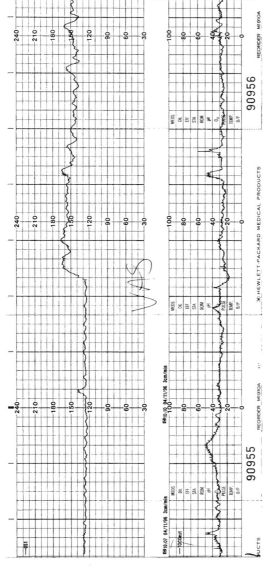

**FIGURE 2–3.** This reactive NST also shows a transition from the nonreactive state (first half of tracing), in which there are no movements and low FHR variability. The onset of normal FHR variability, accelerations, and fetal activity (spikes on lower channel) correspond to VAS. The initial quiet state of the fetus does not signify fetal compromise.

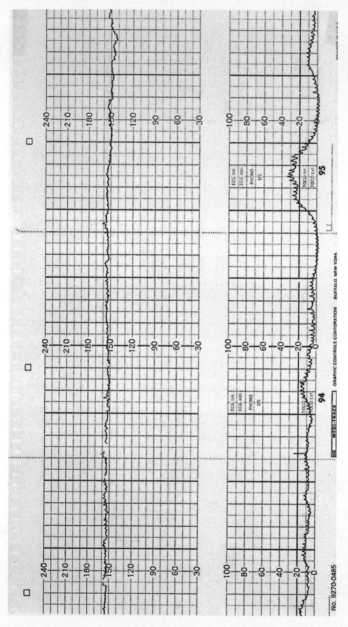

**FIGURE 2–4.**   A nonreactive fetus, with absent movement, virtually absent FHR variability and accelerations, and a suspicious-looking deceleration following the spontaneous uterine contractions in the latter part of the trace. Should this fetus fail to become reactive either spontaneously or following vibroacoustic or manual stimulation, a CST or BPP is indicated.

**3.** Uncertain reactivity: Fewer than two fetal movements in 20 minutes or acceleration of less than 15 beats/min, or for less than 15 seconds; long-term variability amplitude below 6 beats/min; abnormal baseline rate.

A *reactive* test is associated with survival of the fetus for 1 week or more in more than 99 percent of cases.[20] A *nonreactive* test is associated with poor fetal outcome (i.e., perinatal death, low 5-minute Apgar score, late decelerations in labor) in approximately 20 percent of cases. These prediction figures have been obtained from a summary of a large number of patients in reported clinical studies. In an earlier study in which the results of NST were "blinded" (not used in management), the ultimate stillbirth rate of nonreactive fetuses was 26 percent.

Because of the high false-positive rate (80 percent) in clinical application of this test, a nonreactive fetus requires further evaluation by means of the BPP or the CST unless contraindicated. The false-positive rate of the CST is only about 50 percent, and that of the BPP is probably less.

For the fetus with *uncertain* reactivity, another NST should be done within hours or days, or should be followed by a BPP or CST, depending on the clinical situation and the obstetrician's judgment. This decision is modified by the degree of abnormality and specific conditions of each case.

## II    CONTRACTION STRESS TESTING

### A    Technique

The patient is placed in the semi-Fowler's position or left lateral tilt to minimize supine hypotension. Blood pressure may be recorded at intervals. Baseline FHR and contraction pattern are determined for 10 minutes prior to any stimulation of contractions.

Common errors are that the tokodynamometer belt is too loose, giving poor contraction tracings, or that the ultrasound transducer is not directed at the fetal heart, yielding a "noisy," poor-quality FHR tracing.

If there are three adequate contractions in a 10-minute period with a good tracing, the test is complete. This is sometimes called a *spontaneous* CST. The most common error in this period is accepting mildly irregular uterine activity, or high-frequency, low-amplitude contractions, for adequate contractions.

If there are no uterine contractions or if there is inadequate frequency of contractions, they can be provoked by either of two methods: breast stimulation or oxytocin infusion. Breast stimulation is carried out by manual nipple stimulation or application of warm packs to the breasts. Such stimulation should be limited to 2 minutes, with a 5-minute interval before restimulation, in order to avoid prolonged contractions and associated fetal bradycardia.[9]

An alternative method of producing adequate uterine contractions is to begin oxytocin infusion via a small scalp vein needle in a hand vein at 1.0 mU $\cdot$ min$^{-1}$. It is rarely necessary to exceed 10 mU $\cdot$ min$^{-1}$. Oxytocin is increased every 15 to 30 minutes until the contraction rate is three in 10 minutes. If there are late decelerations with each contraction even at a lower frequency than this, the test is complete and the result is positive. Otherwise it is necessary to have three recorded contractions in this 10-minutes period, each with a duration of at least 1 minute. An alternative compromise is to write "C" on the patient's chart, signifying a palpated contraction. If there is any doubt about the adequacy of the challenge, the oxytocin infusion should be continued or increased. After an interpretable test result, the oxytocin infusion is discontinued and the patient is kept on the monitor until uterine activity has returned to baseline frequency.

## B  Interpretation

The following are criteria used for interpretation of the CST:

1. Negative CST result: No late decelerations and normal baseline FHR.

2. Positive CST result: Persistent late decelerations with an adequate challenge or persistent late decelerations even with less than three uterine contractions per 10 minutes (Fig. 2–5). A positive CST with accelerations and normal FHR variability has been called a *reactive positive* CST, and that without accelerations or normal FHR variability has been called a *nonreactive positive* CST.

3. Suspicious CST result: Intermittent late decelerations with an adequate challenge; variable decelerations (which may occur in the growth-restricted fetus with oligohydramnios, and may be due to the cord being compressed during contractions because it is unprotected by amniotic fluid); abnormal baseline FHR (i.e., less than 110 or more than 160 beats/min).

4. Unsatisfactory CST result: Poor-quality recording, perhaps due to maternal obesity or excessive fetal movement; inability to achieve three contractions in 10 minutes.

A fifth type of result, hyperstimulation CST, occurs when late decelerations or prolonged decelerations occur with excessive uterine activity (i.e., contractions closer than every 2 minutes or longer than 90 seconds in duration).

A negative CST result is associated with fetal survival for 1 week in more than 99 percent of cases.[6, 20]

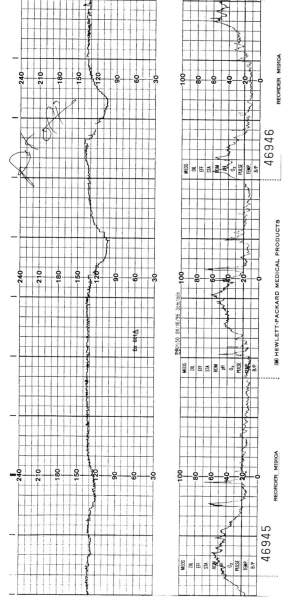

**FIGURE 2–5.** A positive CST, with three late decelerations following each of three oxytocin-induced uterine contractions. The mother noted decreased fetal movement during the preceeding day, and had a nonreactive NST. Her prenatal course was normal except for mild labile hypertension not requiring treatment. She was delivered by cesarean section, and the 2545-g normal-appearing newborn had Apgar scores of 3 (1 minute), 6 (5 minutes), and 7 (10 minutes). Umbilical arterial pH was 6.85, carbon dioxide tension was 99 mmHg, and base excess was $-14$ mEq $\cdot$ l$^{-1}$. No reason was evident for the fetal acidemia, but the newborn did well.

A positive CST result has been associated with poor fetal outcome (i.e., perinatal death, low 5-minute Apgar score, or late decelerations in labor) in approximately 50 percent of cases, in a summary of numerous clinical surveys. In several early studies in which results of the testing were not used to determine management, the ultimate stillbirth rate of fetuses with a positive CST result was 22 percent. However, because of the high false-positive rate, particularly with the positive reactive CST, it is recommended that, if delivery is chosen, such patients be given a trial of labor with optimal FHR monitoring. A positive CST result is prognostically worse if it is accompanied by a nonreactive NST, with absence of both accelerations and FHR variability, and such fetuses are more likely to fail a trial of vaginal delivery.

## C Contraindications

There are certain contraindications (either absolute or relative) to the CST, including previous classical cesarean section, placenta previa, and presence of risk for preterm delivery (e.g., premature rupture of membranes, multiple gestation, incompetent cervix, or treatment for preterm labor).

## III BIOPHYSICAL PROFILE AND ITS MODIFICATION

The BPP has been reported to have a lower false-abnormal rate than either the NST or the CST.[12, 13] However, it has not generally been accepted as the prime means of fetal surveillance, and most clinicians use it to follow up on a nonreactive NST or to clarify the significance of a suspicious or positive CST.

## A Technique

The BPP has five components. It must be done in conjunction with real-time ultrasound. The requirements for maximum scoring, and therefore a well-oxygenated fetus, are as follows:

1. A reactive NST.
2. Presence of fetal breathing movements.
3. Presence of fetal body movements.
4. Fetal tone, including an episode of extension of extremities and return to the flexed position.
5. Adequate amniotic fluid volume.

## B  Interpretation

Points from 0 to 2 are given for each factor. The lower the score, the more likely the fetus is to be compromised. Criteria used at the University of California, San Francisco, are shown in Table 2–1.

Table 2–2 shows a proposed management scheme modified from Manning et al.[13]

## C  Amniotic Fluid Index

The amniotic fluid index (AFI) is a semiquantitative technique used for evaluating amniotic fluid volume.[14, 19] The uterus is divided into four quadrants, with the linea nigra and the umbilicus serving as the dividing points. A linear ultrasound transducer is placed along the patient's longitudinal axis and perpendicular to the floor. Each quadrant is scanned using this technique and the vertical diameter in centimeters of the largest pocket

**TABLE 2–1.    Biophysical Profile Scoring**

|  | Normal (score = 2) | Abnormal (score = 0) |
| --- | --- | --- |
| Fetal breathing movements (FBM) | One or more episodes of FBM (or hiccoughs) of ≥30 sec duration in 20 min | <30 sec of sustained FBM |
| Fetal movements (FM) | Three or more discrete body or limb movements (simultaneous limb and trunk movements are counted as a single movement) in 20 min | No more than two episodes of FM |
| Fetal tone | One or more episodes of active extension with rapid return to flexion of fetal limb(s), trunk, or hand in 20 min | Either slow extension with return to partial flexion or movement of limb in full extension or absent fetal movement |
| Reactive FHR | Two or more accelerations of ≥15 beats/min peak amplitude lasting ≥15 sec at the baseline in 20 min, and decelerations absent | Fewer than two accelerations, or accelerations <15 beats/min peak, or <15 sec duration in 20 min, or decelerations |
| Amniotic fluid index (AFI) | AFI >5.0 | AFI ≤5.0 |

**TABLE 2–2.    Biophysical Profile Scoring and a Suggested Management Scheme**

| Score | Management |
|-------|------------|
| 10 | Repeat weekly |
|    | Repeat twice weekly if >42 weeks or diabetic |
| 8  | Repeat weekly |
|    | Repeat twice weekly if >42 weeks or diabetic |
|    | Consider delivery if oligohydramnios present |
| 6  | Repeat test in 24 hr |
|    | Consider delivery if oligohydramnios present, or score 6 persists at advanced gestational age |
| 4  | Deliver, unless very immature |
|    | If <28 weeks, repeat in 24 hr or less |
| 2  | Test for 120 min |
|    | Deliver as for score 4 |

Modified from Manning FA, Morrison I, Lange IR, et al. Fetal assessment based on fetal biophysical profile scoring: Experience in 12,620 referred high-risk pregnancies. I. Perinatal mortality by frequency and etiology. Am J Obstet Gynecol 1985; 151:343–355.

containing no greater than 50 percent umbilical cord in each quadrant is measured. The sum of the numbers represents the total AFI.

Results are defined as:

| ≤5 | Oligohydramnios |
|------|------|
| >5 to 24 | Normal |
| >24 | Polyhydramnios |

A number of perinatologists are now using a modified BPP, which includes the NST and AFI. When normal, these tests are probably as predictive of good outcome as the full BPP, and are far less time consuming.[5, 16]

---

# IV    ACCURACY OF TESTS

The rates of false-negative and false-positive tests for the various approaches are given in Table 2–3. The data are gathered from various sources, and the accuracy of tests shows some variation, although the accuracy is likely to be better in expert hands.

The false-positive rate has its own hazards, because inappropriately early application of these tests (i.e., in the absence of appropriate indications) may precipitate early delivery and the risks of iatrogenic prematurity.

TABLE 2–3.   **Accuracy of Antepartum Testing Methods**

|  | Nonstress Test | Contraction Stress Test | Modified Biophysical Profile | Biophysical Profile |
|---|---|---|---|---|
| False negative[a] (per 1000) | 3.2 | 0.4 | 0.8 | 0.6 |
| False positive[b] (percent) | 80 | 50 | 60 | 41 |

[a]A false-negative test is fetal death within a week of a normal test, excluding that due to congenital anomalies and unrelated causes.

[b]A false-positive test is birth of a nonasphyxiated fetus following labor despite an "abnormal" test.

See text for sources of data.

 PROTOCOL FOR TESTING: DIAGNOSTIC CONDITIONS AND FREQUENCY

At the University of California, San Francisco, the basic formal testing scheme is the NST and AFI. On occasion the NST alone may suffice. Antenatal testing begins at different gestational ages depending on the maternal and/or fetal condition. It is started either when the condition is recognized [e.g., suspected or actual intrauterine growth restriction (IUGR)] or at specific times (e.g., the postdate pregnancy). For other conditions (e.g., history of late unexplained intrauterine fetal demise) it usually begins in the mid third trimester, about 34 to 36 weeks. The following are some guidelines for testing in specific maternal and fetal conditions.

- Postdate pregnancy: Twice weekly, beginning at 41½ weeks.
- Decreased fetal movement: May only require single test if the NST and AFI are normal and fetal movement returns.
- Hypertensive diseases:

  1. Preeclampsia: weekly or more frequently depending on severity of disease, beginning when recognized.
  2. Chronic hypertension with IUGR: test as per IUGR.
  3. Chronic hypertension without superimposed preeclampsia with normal fetal growth: no formal testing.

- Diabetes mellitus:

  1. Insulin treated without complications, normoglycemic (fasting blood glucose below 100 mg $\cdot$ dl$^{-1}$, postprandial blood glucoses below 130 mg $\cdot$ dl$^{-1}$): weekly, beginning at 36 weeks; if insulin treated before pregnancy, weekly, beginning at 32 weeks.
  2. Insulin treated without complications, but with poor control: weekly, beginning at 32 weeks; twice weekly, beginning at least by 36 weeks.
  3. Insulin treated with complications (e.g., poor fetal growth, vascular disease): beginning when conditions recognized, or by 32 weeks.
  4. Diet-treated glucose intolerance of pregnancy without complications, normoglycemic: no formal testing.

- Intrauterine growth restriction below 10th percentile: twice weekly (or more frequently), beginning when recognized. For suspected IUGR, confirm with ultrasound measurements before testing.
- History of previous unexplained third-trimester intrauterine fetal demise: weekly, beginning at time of prior loss, or by 36 weeks.
- Active substance abuse: weekly. Often these patients have other problems warranting surveillance and testing may improve compliance.
- Increased maternal serum α-fetoprotein (MSAFP) with normal amniocentesis: weekly, beginning at 34 weeks.
- Twins with discordant growth: twice weekly or more frequently as indicated. Discordance is generally considered to be greater than 20 percent discrepancy.
- Preterm premature rupture of membranes (hospitalized): initially may need daily testing (generally BPP) but if stable may need less frequent surveillance.
- Systemic lupus erythematosis, with antinuclear antibody titer above 1/80, or antiphospholipid antibody syndrome: weekly or more frequently, beginning at 34 weeks.
- Oligohydramnios: twice weekly or more frequently, beginning when recognized.
- Rh isoimmunization in the presence of erythroblastosis: weekly or as indicated, beginning at onset of disease.
- Hyperthyroidism: if uncontrolled, weekly, beginning at 32 weeks.
- Cholestasis of pregnancy, with objective evidence: weekly, beginning when recognized.
- Severe polyhydramnios: weekly, beginning when recognized.

- There are many conditions which, when seen alone, may not necessitate antepartum testing. Some examples include well-controlled asthma, advanced maternal age, simple scleroderma, smoking, inactive substance abuse, seizure disorders, noncyanotic maternal heart or lung disease, fetal cardiac problems, omphalocele, decreased MSAFP, and irregularly irregular fetal cardiac arrhythmias.

## VI GUIDELINES FOR FOLLOW-UP OF ABNORMAL TESTING

### A Biophysical Profile

**1.** A nonreactive NST is followed by BPP.

**2.** Guidelines for BPP score:

| | |
|---|---|
| 8 to 10 | Repeat NST/AFI per schedule |
| 6 | Repeat usually 24 hours or less |
| 0 to 4 | Consider for delivery |

### B Contraction Stress Test (Breast Stimulation or Oxytocin)

**1.** May be used as follow-up to NST with suspected decelerations.

**2.** May be used before certain inductions (e.g., prostaglandin gel with decreased AFI).

## VII DOPPLER VELOCIMETRY

This technique is described in Chapter 4. The normal value of the systolic:diastolic (S:D) ratio in the umbilical artery after 30 weeks gestation is less than 3. Values above this represent increases in placental impedance, and correlate with IGUR. Increasing severity of the condition, and increasing impedance, correlate with loss of diastolic flow, and eventually reversed diastolic flow.

Numerous studies have shown that increased S:D ratios or other indices of impedance correlate with fetal morbidity and death.[1] Despite the fact that growth restriction is associated with increased resistance in the umbilical artery, it is neither sensitive nor highly predictive of IUGR. The use of Doppler velocimetry with the other tests of fetal status which appear to be measures of adequacy of fetal oxygenation (NST, CST, BPP) was not shown to be efficacious.[10] The concept that Doppler velocimetry is a placental test rather than a fetal test may have merit,[2] but this implies universal screening, with consequent logistic and economic considerations. It is thus not surprising that the current role of Doppler velocimetry in clinical practice is unclear.[3]

Current conclusions with regard to the use of Doppler velocimetry are as follows:

1. Doppler velocimetry may be useful in raising a recommendation for further testing, which might signify inadequate oxygenation, dysmorphology, or autosomal trisomy.

2. Absent or reversed diastolic flow in the umbilical artery is the most predictive of morbidity and mortality. However, when current noninvasive techniques of fetal assessment (NST, CST, BPP) are available and used, the addition of Doppler velocimetry has not been demonstrated to improve perinatal outcome.

Some cases in which Doppler velocimetry may be useful are:

1. When other tests are unavailable, or other tests are unreliable.

2. Unknown dates in the presence of discordant biometry.

3. When other evaluations of fetal status are borderline.

## REFERENCES

1. Alfirevic Z, Neilson JP. Doppler ultrasonography in high-risk pregnancies: Systematic review with meta-analysis. Am J Obstet Gynecol 1995; 172:1379–1387.

2. Divon MY. Umbilical artery Doppler velocimetry: Clinical utility in high-risk pregnancies. Am J Obstet Gynecol 1996; 174:10–14.

3. Doran JC, Harper H. Where are we with Doppler? Br J Obstet Gynaecol 1994; 101:190–191.

4. Druzin ML. Antepartum fetal heart rate monitoring. State of the art. Clin Perinatol 1989; 16:627–642.

5. Eden R, Seifert L, Kodack L, et al. A modified biophysical profile for antenatal fetal surveillance. Obstet Gynecol 1988; 71:365–369.

6. Evertson LR, Gauthier RJ, Collea JV. Fetal demise following negative contraction stress test. Obstet Gynecol 1978; 51:671–673.

7. Freeman RK, Anderson G, Dorchester W. A prospective multi-institutional study of

antepartum fetal heart rate monitoring. II. Contraction stress test versus nonstress test for primary surveillance. Am J Obstet Gynecol 1982; 143:778–781.

8. Grant A, Elbourne D. Movement counting for assessment of fetal wellbeing. In Chalmers I, Enkin M, Krerse MJ, eds. Effective Care in Pregnancy and Childbirth. Oxford University Press, Oxford, 1989, pp. 440–454.

9. Huddleston JF, Sutliff G, Robinson D. Contraction stress test by intermittent nipple stimulation. Obstet Gynecol 1984; 63:669–673.

10. Johnstone FD, Prescott R, Hoskins P, et al. The effect of introduction of umbilical Doppler recordings to obstetric practice. Br J Obstet Gynaecol 1993; 100:733–738.

11. Keegan KA, Paul RH. Antepartum fetal heart rate testing. IV. The nonstress test as a primary approach. Am J Obstet Gynecol 1980; 136:75–80.

12. Manning FA, Morrison I, Harman CR, Menticoglou SM. The abnormal fetal biophysical profile score. V. Predictive accuracy according to score composition. Am J Obstet Gynecol 1990; 162:918–924.

13. Manning FA, Morrison I, Lange IR, et al. Fetal assessment based on fetal biophysical profile scoring: Experience in 12,620 referred high-risk pregnancies. I. Perinatal mortality by frequency and etiology. Am J Obstet Gynecol 1985; 151:343–355.

14. Moore TR, Cayle JE. The amniotic fluid index in normal human pregnancy. Am J Obstet Gynecol 1990; 162:1168–1173.

15. Moore TR, Piacquadio K. A prospective evaluation of fetal movement screening to reduce the incidence of antepartum fetal death. Am J Obstet Gynecol 1989; 160:1075–1080.

16. Nageotte MP, Towers CV, Asrat T, Freeman RK. Perinatal outcome with the modified biophysical profile. Am J Obstet Gynecol 1994; 170:1672–1676.

17. Neldam S. Fetal movements as an indicator of fetal well-being. Dan Med Bull 1983; 30:274–280.

18. Nijuis JG, Prechtl HFR, Martin CB Jr, Bots RSGM. Are there behavioural states in the human fetus? Early Hum Dev 1982; 6:177–195.

19. Phelan JP, Ohn MO, Smith CV, et al. Amniotic fluid index measurements during pregnancy. J Reprod Med 1987; 32:603–604.

20. Schifrin BS. The rationale for antepartum fetal heart rate monitoring. J Reprod Med 1979; 23:213–221.

21. Smith CV, Phelan JP, Platt LD, et al. Fetal acoustic stimulation testing. II. A randomized clinical comparison with the nonstress test. Am J Obstet Gynecol 1986; 155:131–134.

22. Thacker SB, Berkelman RL. Assessing the diagnostic accuracy and efficacy of selected antepartum fetal surveillance techniques. Obstet Gynecol 1986; 41:121–130.

# Part Two

# PHYSIOLOGY

# ■ *Chapter Three*

# Uteroplacental Circulation and Respiratory Gas Exchange

The placenta is a union of maternal and fetal tissues for purposes of physiologic exchange. Because the ultimate cause of most stillbirths and many depressed fetuses is intrauterine asphyxia, the factors responsible for adequacy of placental function, particularly respiratory gas exchange, assume great importance.

## I  PLACENTAL ANATOMY AND CIRCULATION

The human placenta is described as a villous hemochorial type. The villi are projections of fetal tissue surrounded by chorion that are exposed to circulating maternal blood. The chorion is the outermost fetal tissue layer. At term the human placenta weighs about 500 g and is disc shaped, with a diameter of approximately 20 cm and a thickness of 3 cm. The fetal:placental weight ratio is normally approximately 6:1 at term. Prior to this the placenta is relatively heavier and the ratio is less (e.g., 3:1 at 30 weeks' gestation).

Circulation of blood through the placenta is illustrated in Figure 3–1. The maternal blood is carried initially in the uterine arteries, and these ultimately divide into spiral arteries in the basal plate. Blood is spurted, probably under arterial pressure, from these arteries into the intervillous space. It traverses upward toward the chorionic plate, passing fetal villi, and finally drains back to veins in the basal plate. It is likely that throughout this passage past the villi the maternal blood is exchanging substances with fetal blood within the villi.

The fetal circulation within the placenta is quite different. Blood is carried into the placenta by two umbilical arteries that successively divide into smaller vessels within the fetal villi. Ultimately, capillaries traverse the tips of

**27**

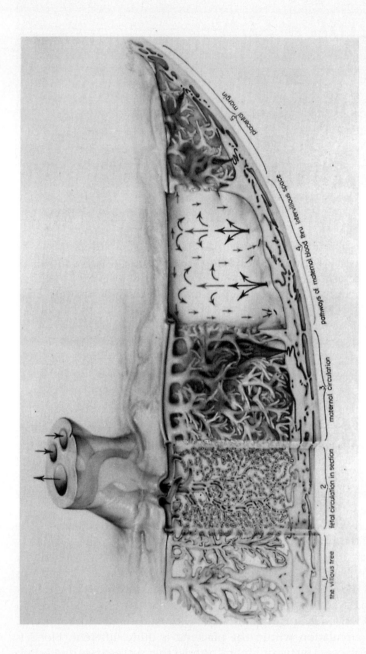

**FIGURE 3–1.** The circulation of blood in the primate placenta. Fetal circulation is shown in the two panels at left and in the umbilical cord above. The right panels show the maternal blood spurting from spiral arteries in the basal area through the intervillous space. The blood passes fetal villi, exchanges substances with fetal blood within the villi, and ultimately drains into veins in the basal area. (Drawing by Ranice W. Crosby for the late Dr. Elizabeth M. Ramsey. Reprinted by courtesy of the Carnegie Institution of Washington, D.C.)

the fetal villi, and it is at this point that exchange occurs with maternal blood within the intervillous space. The blood is finally collected into a single umbilical vein in the umbilical cord, and this carries the nutrient-rich and waste-poor blood to the fetus.

Fetal and maternal blood are separated by three microscopic tissue layers in the human placenta. The first layer is the fetal trophoblast, which consists of cytotrophoblast and syncytiotrophoblast. The syncytiotrophoblast is the metabolically active part of the placenta rich in receptors to many factors, channels, enzymes, and organelles, and the region where much of the endocrine function of the placenta occurs.[6] The other tissue layers are fetal connective tissue, which serves to support the villi, and the endothelium of fetal capillaries (Fig. 3–2).

The quantitative relationship of fetal and maternal blood flow and relative concentrations of substances at any one point in the human placenta are quite complex. The relative rates of blood flow in various areas of the placenta are quite variable, and there is a continually changing concentration of nutrients and waste materials in various areas of the placenta as exchange occurs.[10]

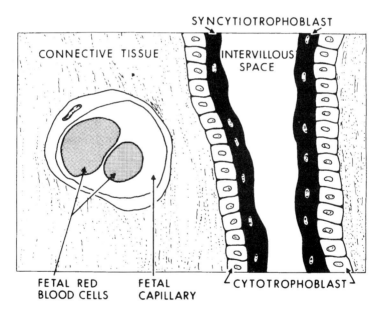

**FIGURE 3–2.** Drawing from an electron micrograph of a cross-section through parts of two fetal villi, showing tissue layers that separate fetal and maternal blood in the human placenta. The cytotrophoblastic layer is much less distinct in the third trimester than is depicted here.

# II  MECHANISMS OF EXCHANGE

Substances are exchanged across the placental membrane by five mechanisms: diffusion, active transport, bulk flow, pinocytosis, and breakage.[6, 8]

## A  Diffusion

Diffusion is a physicochemical process in which no energy is required and substances pass from one area to another on the basis of a concentration gradient. The respiratory gases oxygen and carbon dioxide, the fatty acids, and the smaller ions (e.g., $Na^+$ and $Cl^-$) are transported by this mechanism.

Facilitated diffusion describes the mechanism of passage of glucose and some other carbohydrates. With this mechanism substances still pass down a concentration gradient, but the rate of passage is greater than can be explained by the gradient alone. Carrier molecules are involved, and there is a need for energy expenditure.

## B  Active Transport

Active transport allows for the passage of substances through channels in a direction against the concentration gradient. Energy is required, there are carrier molecules involved, and active transport is subject to inhibition by certain metabolites. The amino acids, water-soluble vitamins, and some of the larger ions (e.g., $Ca^{2+}$ and $Fe^{2+}$) are transported by this mechanism.

## C  Bulk Flow

Bulk flow describes the passage of substances due to a hydrostatic or osmotic gradient. Water is transported by this mechanism and may also carry some solutes with it under the influence of this mechanism.

## D  Pinocytosis

Some large molecules, such as the immune globulins, are transported by being enclosed in small vesicles consisting of cell membranes. These are pinched off on one side of the placenta and traverse to the other side, where their contents are released.

## E  Breakage

The delicate, filmy villi may at times break off within the intervillous space, and the contents may be extruded into the maternal circulation. It is also thought that maternal intravascular contents may be taken up by the fetal circulation at times. The most important result of this is seen when fetal Rh-positive red cells are deposited in the vascular system of an Rh-negative mother, resulting in isoimmunization and subsequent erythroblastosis fetalis.

---

# III DIFFUSION

When limitations of placental transfer occur in the human, they usually are first recognized as limitations of those substances that are exchanged by diffusion. For example, an acute decrease in placental function limits passage of oxygen to and carbon dioxide from the fetus, resulting in fetal asphyxia. A more chronic decrease in placental function may result in limitation of substances necessary for growth (e.g., carbohydrates), thus giving rise to a fetus that is growth retarded. Hence, the process of diffusion is examined in some detail.

Fick's diffusion equation describes the physicochemical process:

$$\text{Rate of transfer} = \frac{\text{concentration gradient} \times \text{area} \times \text{permeability}}{\text{membrane thickness}}$$

Each of the factors determining rate of passage of substances by diffusion is considered in turn.

## A Concentration Gradient

The concentration gradient of a substance across the placenta is equal to the difference between the mean maternal blood concentration and the mean fetal blood concentration within each of the exchanging areas. As noted above, however, it is most unlikely that this gradient is constant throughout the placenta because of the placenta's peculiar circulatory anatomy. It probably varies from place to place and also from time to time in any particular area. However, by considering a simplified exchanging membrane with blood flowing in from each side, each of the factors that would affect the concentration gradient can be conceptually discussed (Fig. 3–3). These factors are

1. Concentration of substance in maternal arterial blood.
2. Concentration of substance in fetal arterial blood.
3. Maternal intervillous space blood flow.
4. Fetal–placental blood flow.
5. Diffusing capacity of the placenta for the substance.

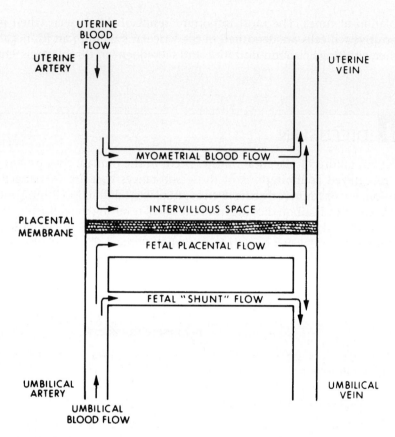

**FIGURE 3–3.** Simplified diagram of pattern of circulation through the placenta.

6. Ratio of maternal to fetal blood flow in exchanging areas. This is analogous to ventilation:perfusion ratios as applied to the lung. Inequalities in the ratio give rise to decreased efficiency of transfer. Exchange of substances is optimal if the flows are evenly matched.

7. Binding of substances to molecules and dissociation rates. Depending on the rate of dissociation, this reaction time could limit the transfer of a substance. This does not appear to be limiting with regard to the dissociation of oxygen and hemoglobin.

8. Geometry of exchanging surfaces with respect to blood flow. If blood flows are traveling in the same direction during exchange the system is called *concurrent*. If the blood flows are traveling in opposite directions the system is called *countercurrent*. This latter system is the most efficient

from the exchange point of view. As can be seen in Figure 3–1, in the human placenta it is unlikely that either of these simplified concepts holds. The human pattern has been described as the *multivillous stream system*.[10] The evaluation of the mean concentration gradient of any nutrient in this system becomes extremely complex.

**9.** The metabolism of the substance. If a substance is consumed within the placenta, its rate of passage across the placenta will not be reflected by the concentration gradient. For example, oxygen is consumed in considerable quantities by the trophoblast and the rate of passage appears to be relatively inefficient when based on oxygen tension gradients alone.

## B Area of the Placenta

The villous surface area of the human term placenta[1, 6] is approximately 11 m². In comparison, the lung has an alveolar surface area of 70 m². The area of actual exchange, the vasculosyncytial membrane—that is, the area where fetal capillaries approach closely enough to the surface to exchange materials with maternal blood—is 1.8 m².

Placental area is decreased in a number of clinical situations. An acute decrease occurs with abruptio placentae. With part of the placenta separated, the fetus does not necessarily expire through asphyxia. Its ability to survive depends on the area lost, and on the placental reserve that existed before the episode of abruption. Some placentas, particularly those in cases of maternal hypertension or those that have infarcted fibrotic areas, have a reduced area available for exchange and, hence, lowered reserve. Thus, the placenta of a mother with long-term hypertension is likely to be smaller than expected, as is the fetus. The infarctions are thought to be caused by maternal arteriolar deficiencies giving rise to devitalization of certain cotyledonary areas, resulting in fibrosis of the villi. Additionally, in certain cases of intrauterine infection or congenital defects, the placentas are decreased in size and area. Large placentas are found in certain diabetics and in erythroblastosis fetalis. In the former case, it is not certain whether the increased area improves the transfer of nutrients to the fetus. In the latter case, most of the increased placental mass is thought to be hydropic in origin and, hence, is unlikely to improve the exchange characteristics of the placenta.

## C Permeability of the Placental Membrane

The permeability of a membrane to a substance depends on characteristics both of the membrane and of the substance that is exchanging. The units for permeability can be found by a transposition of Fick's diffusion equation.

There are three major determinants of permeability:

1. Molecular size. A molecular weight of 1000 is a rough dividing line between those substances that cross the placenta by diffusion and those that are relatively impermeable by diffusion. Below a molecular weight of 1000 the rate of passage of the molecule is related to its weight unless other properties (see below) prevent or hasten rate of passage. A common clinical example is found in cases in which it is necessary to anticoagulate a pregnant woman. If one uses heparin, with a molecular weight above 6000, one does not concomitantly heparinize the fetus. However, with the use of warfarin (Coumadin), with a molecular weight of 330, the fetus will also be anticoagulated. This is considered undesirable, particularly in the intrapartum period, when fetal bleeding may occur. Also, warfarin may have some teratogenic effects in the first trimester.

2. Lipid solubility. A lipid-soluble substance traverses the placenta more rapidly than one that is not lipid soluble.

3. Electrical charge. This deters the passage of a substance across the placenta. For example, succinylcholine, commonly used during balanced anesthesia, is highly ionized and is poorly diffusable across the placenta despite its molecular weight of 361. Thiopental, with a molecular weight of 264, is lipid soluble, relatively un-ionized, and moves very rapidly into the fetal circulation.

Substances are classified into those in which the rate of passage is either *permeability limited* or *flow limited*.[9] A substance that is poorly permeable is limited in its rate of passage across the placenta by permeability and not by rates of blood flow. Hence, increasing the rate of blood flow will not improve its rate of passage much at all. The majority of biologic molecules are limited in their rate of passage across the placenta by resistance to diffusion. However, substances that are highly permeable are limited by the rate of blood flow. Oxygen and carbon dioxide are examples of this. Decreasing the rate of blood flow has a relatively strong influence on decreasing the rate of exchange.

## D  Diffusion Distance

The average distance for diffusion across the placenta[1] has been measured as approximately 3.5 μm. This contrasts with the much smaller distance from alveolus to pulmonary capillary in the lung (0.5 μm). The diffusion distance decreases as the placenta matures, but it is not clear whether this improves the placenta's characteristics for exchange. The distance is increased in several conditions, such as erythroblastosis fetalis and congenital syphilis. This increased distance is probably due to villous edema and presumably decreases the organ's efficiency for exchange. Fibrous or calcific deposits in the placental vasculature, such as are found in diabetes mellitus or preeclampsia, presumably increase diffusion distance.

# IV UTERINE BLOOD FLOW

Because uterine blood flow is one of the prime determinants of passage of a number of critical substances across the placenta, its characteristics and the factors affecting it are discussed. Uterine blood flow rises progressively throughout pregnancy and in the term fetus is approximately 700 ml • min$^{-1}$. This represents about 10% of the cardiac output. Approximately 70 to 90 percent of the uterine blood flow passes through the intervillous space, and the remainder largely supplies the myometrium.

The uterine vascular bed is thought to be almost maximally dilated under normal conditions, with little capacity to dilate further.[2] It is not autoregulated, so flow is proportional to the mean perfusion pressure. However, it is capable of marked vasoconstriction by $\alpha$-adrenergic action. It is not responsive to changes in respiratory gas tensions. The uterine blood flow is determined by the following relationship:

$$\text{Uterine blood flow} = \frac{\text{uterine arterial pressure} - \text{uterine venous pressure}}{\text{uterine vascular resistance}}$$

Hence, any factor affecting any of the three values on the right side of the above relationship will alter uterine blood flow. A number of causes of decreased uterine blood flow are shown in Table 3–1.

Uterine contractions are thought to decrease uterine blood flow because of increased uterine venous pressure brought about by increased intramural pressure of the uterus (Fig. 3–4). There may also be a decrease in uterine arterial diameter with contractions. Uterine hypertonus causes a decreased uterine blood flow through the same mechanism.

In sheep it has been shown that, if uterine arterial perfusion pressure is altered without changing the resistance of the uterine vascular bed, there is a direct relationship between uterine blood flow and the pressure.[2] Hence, hypotension through any of the mechanisms noted in Table 3–1 will cause a decrease in blood flow.

In the case of maternal arterial hypertension it is likely that there is a concomitant increased vascular resistance that is shared by the uterine vascular bed. This therefore results in a decrease in uterine blood flow. Either endogenous or exogenous vasoconstriction results in decreased blood flow because of increased uterine vascular resistance.

**TABLE 3–1.  Factors Causing Decreased Uterine Blood Flow**

**Uterine contractions**

**Hypertonus**
 Abruptio placentae
 Tetanic contraction
 Overstimulation with oxytocin

**Hypotension**
 Sympathetic block
 Hypovolemic shock
 Supine hypotensive syndrome

**Hypertension**
 Essential
 Preeclampsia

**Vasoconstriction, endogenous**
 Sympathetic discharge
 Adrenal medullary activity

**Vasoconstrictors, exogenous**
 Most sympathomimetics (α-adrenergic effects)
 Exception is ephedrine (primarily β-adrenergic effects)

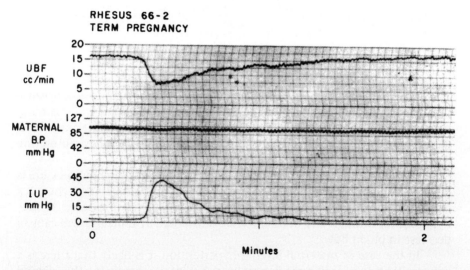

**FIGURE 3–4.**   Uterine contraction in a pregnant monkey, showing the concomitant "mirror image" decrease in uterine blood flow. This phenomenon probably occurs with every contraction in every woman in labor. UBF, uterine blood flow; measured by electromagnetic flow meter. IUP, intrauterine pressure. (From Greiss F Jr. Uterine blood flow during labor. Clin Obstet Gynecol 1968; 11:96. Used by permission.)

There are few useful means of increasing uterine blood flow in cases in which it is known to be less than optimal. The most important clinical considerations are the avoidance or correction of factors responsible for an acute decrease in blood flow (e.g., excessive uterine activity or maternal hypotension).

Some of the β-mimetic agents that are used as uterine relaxants for preterm labor may increase uterine blood flow, but this effect, if any, is small and may only be a result of decreased uterine tonus. There are a number of experimental means of increasing uterine blood flow, sometimes transiently, but these have no place clinically. Examples of such treatments include estrogens, acetylcholine, nitroglycerine, cyanide, ischemia, and mild hypoxia, the latter either acute or chronic.[4]

Clinically, it has been suspected for many years that maternal bed rest may improve the outcome in fetal growth retardation. This may be due to an overall higher uterine blood flow throughout the day when the patient is reclining, compared to the active, ambulatory state.

## V  OXYGEN TRANSFER TO THE FETUS

It is likely that many stillbirths and cases of fetal depression are the result of inadequate exchange of the respiratory gases. Oxygen has the lowest storage: utilization ratio of all nutrients in the fetus. From animal experimentation it can be calculated that in a term fetus the quantity of oxygen is approximately 42 ml and the normal oxygen consumption is approximately $21 \text{ ml} \cdot \text{min}^{-1}$.[3] This means that, in theory, the fetus has a 2-minute supply of oxygen. However, fetuses do not consume the total quantity of oxygen in their body within 2 minutes, nor do they expire after this time. In fact, irreversible brain damage does not occur until about 10 minutes have elapsed.[11] This is because the fetus has a number of important compensatory mechanisms that enable it to survive on a lesser quantity of oxygen for longer periods. Clinical situations in which there is total cessation of oxygen delivery are rare. These include sudden total abruption of the placenta or complete umbilical cord compression, generally after prolapse of the cord.

It is known from animal experimentation that the compensations that occur in the hypoxic fetus are (a) redistribution of blood flow favoring vital organs, including heart, brain, adrenal glands, and placenta; (b) decreased total oxygen consumption (e.g., with moderate hypoxia the fetal oxygen consumption drops to 50% of the normal level); and (c) dependence of certain vascular beds on anaerobic metabolism. These compensatory mechanisms appear to be initiated with mild to moderate hypoxia and result in the maintenance of oxygen supply to vital organs during times of oxygen limitation.[3]

It is of value to examine the factors that determine oxygen transfer from mother to fetus (Table 3–2). Because the transfer of oxygen to the fetus is dependent on rates of blood flow and not limitations to diffusion, the respective blood flow on each side of the placenta assumes major importance for maintenance of fetal oxygenation. As noted in Figure 3–4, small reductions in uterine blood flow normally occur with uterine contractions, and probably result in a small reduction in fetal oxygen tension. This has been demonstrated in the sheep (Fig. 3–5), and probably also occurs in humans. Note that the decrease in oxygen tension is small, approximately 2 mmHg; this is presumed to be of little consequence to the normal fetus, and to be insufficient to trigger any compensatory mechanisms.

Animal work suggests that in the normal placenta there is a "safety factor" of approximately 50 percent in the uterine blood flow. That is, the uterine blood flow will drop to half its normal value before severe fetal acidosis becomes evident[12] and oxygen uptake declines.[14] Approximately the same effect may occur with less of half of the placental area in abruptio placentae, but this is overshadowed by the deleterious effects of uterine hypertonus, probably because of myometrial irritation from extravasated blood.

The "safety factor" only applies to the normal situation with normal placental reserve and is unlikely to be the case in pathologic situations, such as the infant of the hypertensive mother. In such situations the placental function may be adequate for oxygenation but not for fetal growth, and a growth-retarded infant may result from such a pregnancy. Furthermore, with superimposition of uterine contractions on such a fetus, there may be transient inadequacy of uterine blood flow during the uterine contractions;

**TABLE 3–2.   Factors Determining the Maternal–Fetal Oxygen Transfer**

Intervillous blood flow
Fetal placental blood flow
Oxygen tension in maternal arterial blood
Oxygen tension in fetal arterial blood
Oxygen affinity of maternal blood
Oxygen affinity of fetal blood
Hemoglobin concentration or oxygen capacity of maternal blood
Hemoglobin concentration or oxygen capacity of fetal blood
Maternal and fetal blood pH and partial pressure of carbon dioxide (Bohr effect)
Placental diffusing capacity
Placental vascular geometry
Ratio of maternal to fetal blood flow in exchanging areas
Shunting around exchange sites
Placental oxygen consumption

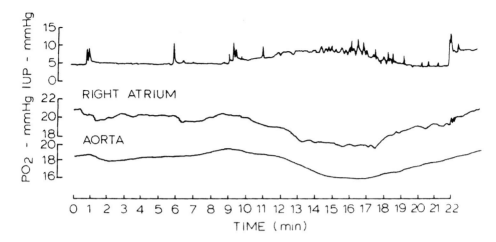

**FIGURE 3–5.** Continuously measured fetal aortic arch and right atrium oxygen pressure during a spontaneously occurring prelabor uterine contraction in a sheep. (From Jansen CA, Krane EJ, Thomas AL, Beck NF, Lowe KC, Joyce P, Parr M, Nathanielsz PW. Continuous variability of fetal $pO_2$ in the chronically catheterized fetal sheep. Am J Obstet Gynecol 1979; 134:776–783. Used by permission.)

this may be recognized by responses of the fetal heart rate (i.e., late decelerations).

Additional important determinants of fetal oxygenation include oxygen tension in maternal arterial and fetal arterial blood. In general, maternal arterial oxygen tension depends on adequate ventilation and pulmonary integrity. Disruptions of this function are relatively rare in obstetrics, although they can occur with pulmonary diseases such as asthma, in cases of congestive heart failure, or in mothers with congenital cardiac defects.

The oxygen affinity and oxygen capacity of maternal and fetal blood are also important determinants of fetal oxygen transfer. The amount of oxygen carried by the blood depends on the partial pressure of oxygen in the blood and the affinity of hemoglobin for oxygen. The degree to which hemoglobin takes up oxygen is depicted on the oxygen dissociation curve. Figure 3–6 depicts oxygen dissociation curves of maternal and fetal blood at a constant temperature (37°C) and pH (7.4). It relates the percentage of saturation of the hemoglobin with oxygen to the partial pressure to which the blood is exposed. In Figure 3–6, the maternal curve is to the right of the fetal curve. The fetal blood is said to have a higher affinity for oxygen than does the maternal blood. As shown in the diagram, at a partial pressure of oxygen of 30 mmHg, for example, maternal blood is 57 percent saturated with oxygen, whereas at the same partial pressure, fetal blood is approximately 74 percent saturated. Because there is more oxygen in fetal blood than in maternal blood, it would

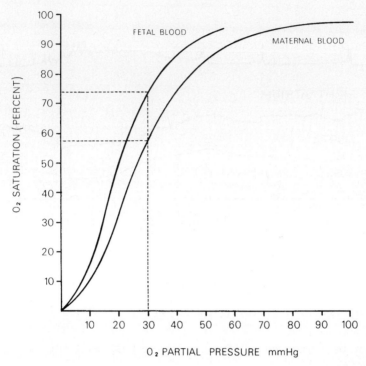

**FIGURE 3–6.** Oxygen dissociation curves of maternal and fetal blood. The vertical broken line illustrates the higher oxygen affinity of fetal blood. Fetal blood is more highly saturated with oxygen than is maternal blood at the same oxygen partial pressure.

appear that oxygen is traveling against a concentration gradient; however, this is not so, as the concentration of oxygen that determines the rate of passage of oxygen is that found in plasma, and not that bound to hemoglobin. Plasma oxygen concentration is related to oxygen tension rather than to total oxygen concentration.

The quantity of oxygen carried in the blood is also a function of the oxygen capacity of the blood, which is directly related to hemoglobin concentration. Each gram of hemoglobin combines with 1.34 ml of oxygen, and there is normally a difference in the hemoglobin concentrations of maternal and fetal blood. Maternal blood has a hemoglobin concentration of approximately 12 g $\cdot$ dl$^{-1}$, whereas the hemoglobin concentration of fetal blood is approximately 15 g $\cdot$ dl$^{-1}$. This difference means that the fetus has an added advantage.

In Figure 3–7, the difference in oxygen capacity has been incorporated into the vertical axis, so that oxygen content is related to the partial pressure of oxygen in maternal and fetal blood. It should be noted that once again at the same partial pressure (30 mm Hg), the fetal blood contains almost 15 ml $\cdot$ dl$^{-1}$ (milliliters per 100 ml of blood) of oxygen, whereas that of the mother has approximately 9 ml $\cdot$ dl$^{-1}$. The added advantage to fetal oxygenation of the higher hemoglobin content of fetal blood thus is demonstrated.

The position of the oxygen dissociation curve is altered by changes in the pH. This phenomenon is termed the *Bohr effect*. At acidic pHs, the curve shifts to the right; at alkaline pHs, it shifts to the left. Any factor that tends to exaggerate the difference between the two oxygen dissociation curves will be advantageous to oxygen exchange, because it increases the gradient. As maternal blood gives up oxygen and takes up carbon dioxide in the placenta, the maternal curve shifts to the right. The reverse happens in fetal blood: It gives up carbon dioxide to maternal blood and becomes more alkaline, which

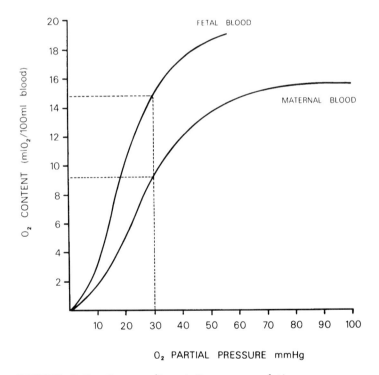

**FIGURE 3–7.** Oxygen dissociation curves relating oxygen content of blood to oxygen partial pressure in maternal and fetal blood. This relationship illustrates the even greater oxygen content of fetal blood when the greater hemoglobin content of fetal blood is taken into account.

results in a shift of the curve to the left. These factors facilitate oxygen exchange to the fetus.

The other properties that affect oxygen transfer across the placenta have been discussed in the section on determinants of concentration gradient. These factors include placental diffusing capacity, placental vascular geometry, ratio of maternal to fetal blood flow in the exchanging areas, shunting of blood around exchange sites, and metabolism of oxygen within the placenta.

Oxygen exchange in the human placenta is shown in Figure 3–8. This figure depicts the oxygen dissociation curves of maternal and fetal blood using the hemoglobin concentrations noted previously. Superimposed are points showing the probable values, under normal conditions in late pregnancy, of maternal and fetal oxygen concentrations and tensions at sampling points in

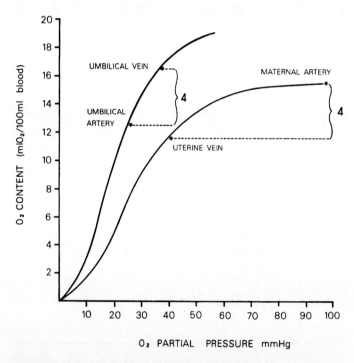

**FIGURE 3–8.** Summary of oxygen exchange in the placenta, showing probable values of oxygen content and partial pressure in the uterine and umbilical arteries and veins in the undisturbed state. Free use has been made of data from chronic preparations in experimental animals. The brackets show the arteriovenous oxygen differences on the maternal and fetal side: 4 ml of oxygen is delivered or given up by each 100 ml of circulating blood.

the four major vessels that supply and drain the placenta. Some error is introduced because blood cannot be sampled before admixture with the shunted blood. It should be noted that the samples from the fetus and the uterine vein are slightly to the right of the oxygen dissociation curves (which have been drawn at a pH of 7.4), because they are generally slightly more acidotic.

Also shown in the diagram are the arteriovenous oxygen differences in the maternal and fetal vessels. The arteriovenous difference (4 ml $\cdot$ dl$^{-1}$) is a measure of the quantity of oxygen taken up or released by each 100 ml of circulating blood through the various organs. These figures are largely estimates taken from fetal scalp blood sampling and data obtained from experimental animals. Values of umbilical arterial and venous blood have been obtained from the relatively undisturbed human fetus, and they are similar to the values shown here.[13] Further aspects of decreased oxygen transfer from the mother to the fetus are considered in Chapter 4.

## VI CARBON DIOXIDE AND ACID-BASE BALANCE

Carbon dioxide crosses the placenta even more readily than does oxygen. In general the determinants for oxygen transfer also apply to carbon dioxide transfer across the placenta. It is limited by rate of blood flow and not by resistance to diffusion. The carbon dioxide tension in fetal blood in the undisturbed state is close to 40 mmHg.[13] It is well known that the maternal arterial carbon dioxide tension is approximately 34 mm Hg, and the mother is in a state of compensated respiratory alkalosis. The pH of fetal blood under undisturbed conditions is probably close to 7.4, and the bicarbonate concentration is close to that in maternal blood.

Bicarbonate and the fixed acids cross the placenta much more slowly than does carbon dioxide; that is, equilibration takes a matter of hours rather than seconds. There is a situation analogous to "respiratory acidosis" that occurs in the fetus when blood flow, either uterine or umbilical, is acutely transiently compromised. In such cases, carbon dioxide tension is elevated and the pH drops, but the metabolic acid-base status remains unchanged. This occurs during severe or profound fetal decelerations (called *variable decelerations*)[5, 7] in association with certain uterine contractions. These acid-base changes are generally rapidly resolved with cessation of the contraction and the deceleration. However, as noted earlier, if there is a significant oxygen lack that is unrelieved, the fetus will decrease its oxygen consumption, redistribute blood flow, and depend partly on anaerobic metabolism to supply its energy needs, albeit with decreased efficiency. Under these conditions, lactate (an end product of anaerobic metabolism) is produced, resulting in a metabolic acidosis. The acidosis may also be aggravated by a combined respiratory acidosis because of retained carbon dioxide. Unlike carbon dioxide, lactate is lost rather slowly from the fetus.

## VII   CLINICAL IMPLICATIONS

Fetal compromise results from a disruption of normal placental exchange mechanisms. With a knowledge of the components involved in exchange of nutrients and waste materials across the placenta, potential problems can be recognized and corrections can be made.

The most important components of placental exchange are the rates of blood flow on each side of the placenta and the area available for exchange. Uterine blood flow will decline in the presence of factors causing decreased perfusion pressure or increased uterine vascular resistance. Common clinical occurrences are hypotension, hypertension, endogenous or exogenous vaso-constriction, and possibly severe psychological stress. The uterine vascular bed, as previously noted, is not autoregulated and has little capacity to dilate further. During labor, it is most likely that the rate of uterine blood flow is the limiting factor in cases of fetal compromise because of the intermittent decline in uterine blood flow with each uterine contraction. In addition, transient or persistent umbilical cord compression may interfere with respiratory gas exchange in the fetus.

## REFERENCES

1. Aherne W, Dunnill MS. Morphometry of the human placenta. Br Med Bull 1966; 22:5–8.

2. Assali NS, Brinkman CR III. The uterine circulation and its control. In Longo LD, Bartels H, eds. Respiratory Gas Exchange and Blood Flow in the Placenta. U.S. Department of Health, Education and Welfare, Washington, DC, 1972, pp. 121–141.

3. Court DJ, Parer JT. Experimental studies in fetal asphyxia and fetal heart rate interpretation. In Nathanielsz PW, Parer JT, eds. Research in Perinatal Medicine (I). Perinatology Press, Ithaca, NY, 1985, pp. 114–164.

4. Greiss F Jr. Concepts of uterine blood flow. In Wynn RM, ed. Obstetrics and Gynecology Annual. Appleton-Century-Crofts, New York, 1973, pp. 55–83.

5. Hon EH, Khazin AF. Biochemical studies of the fetus. I. The fetal pH-measuring system. Obstet Gynecol 1969; 33:219–236.

6. Kaufmann P, Burton G. Anatomy and genesis of the placenta. Chapter 8 in Knobil E, Neill JD, eds. The Physiology of Reproduction. Raven Press, New York, 1994, pp. 441–483.

7. Kubli FW, Hon EH, Khazin AF, Takemura H. Observations on heart rate and pH in the human fetus during labor. Am J Obstet Gynecol 1969; 104:1190–1206.

8. Longo LD. Placental transfer mechanisms—an overview. In Wynn RM, ed. Obstetrics and Gynecology Annual. Appleton-Century-Crofts, New York, 1972, pp. 103–138.

9. Meschia G. Physiology of transplacental diffusion. In Wynn RM, ed. Obstetrics and Gynecology Annual. Appleton-Century-Crofts, New York, 1976, pp. 21–38.

10. Metcalfe J, Bartels H, Moll W. Gas exchange in the pregnant uterus. Physiol Rev 1967; 47:782–838.

11. Myers RE. Two patterns of perinatal brain damage and their conditions of occurrence. Am J Obstet Gynecol 1972; 112:246–276.

12. Parer JT, Behrman RE. The influence of uterine blood flow on the acid-base status of the rhesus monkey. Am J Obstet Gynecol 1970; 107:1241–1249.

13. Soothill PW, Nicolaides KH, Rodeck CH, Campbell S. Effects of gestational age on fetal and intervillous blood gas and acid-base values in human pregnancy. Fetal Therapy 1986; 1:168–175.

14. Wilkening RB, Meschia G. Fetal oxygen uptake, oxygenation and acid-base balance as a function of uterine blood flow. Am J Physiol 1983; 24:H749–H755.

# ■ *Chapter Four*

# Fetal Cardiorespiratory Physiology

## I · ANATOMY OF FETAL CIRCULATION

In the adult, blood travels from the left ventricle to the systemic circulation and is returned to the right side of the heart. From there, it flows through the lungs for reoxygenation. This serial circulatory design is inappropriate for the fetus, because oxygenation occurs in the placenta, and a pair of parallel circulations is present. Fetal circulation is made possible by anatomical "shunts," which normally are closed rapidly at birth, when adult circulation is required.[7]

The fetal circulation is illustrated in Figure 4–1, with approximate values of the percentage of saturation of blood with oxygen in various areas. Most of the physiologic data presented in this section are taken from studies of chronically catheterized, unanesthetized sheep fetuses, because it is rarely possible to obtain extensive data from the human fetus. Although species differences may occur, it is likely that the same general trends and mechanisms apply to the human fetus as apply to the sheep fetus.

Well-oxygenated blood returns from the placenta by way of the umbilical vein (Fig. 4–2). This vein enters the liver, where it joins with the portal venous system. Some of the blood is shunted directly to the inferior vena cava through the ductus venosus, and some traverses the hepatic parenchyma. An average of 50 percent takes the latter path, but the proportion is variable.

The saturation of blood in the inferior vena cava is lower than that in the ductus venosus, because it has mixed with poorly oxygenated blood returning from the lower body. The inferior vena caval blood enters the right atrium, and approximately 40 percent is diverted immediately by way of the

**47**

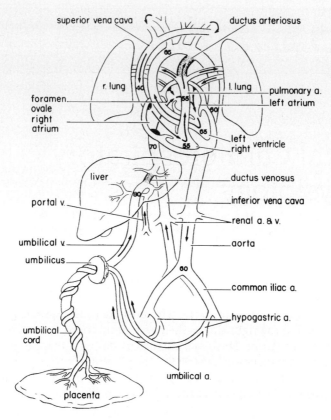

**FIGURE 4–1.** The fetal circulation. Numbers represent approximate values of the percentage of saturation of the blood hemoglobin with oxygen in utero.

foramen ovale (another temporary shunt) to the left atrium. Here it mixes with a relatively small quantity of pulmonary venous blood and enters the left ventricle and then the coronary circulation and the vessels that supply the head, neck, and upper extremities. Hence, the foramen ovale allows relatively well-oxygenated blood to supply two vital structures, the heart and the head.

Blood entering the right atrium from the superior vena cava joins with the remaining 60 percent of inferior vena caval blood and enters the right ventricle (Fig. 4–3). From here, a small proportion enters the pulmonary circulation, but most is shunted from this bed by way of the ductus arteriosus, which joins the descending aorta (Fig. 4–4). Descending aortic blood supplies the gut, kidneys, and lower body and also the umbilical circulation.

# II   DISTRIBUTION OF BLOOD FLOWS

The distribution of blood flows in the fetus generally is described as a percentage of the cardiac output. It is a simple concept in the adult, who has two essentially equal serial circulations, systemic and pulmonary. In the fetus, with two unequal parallel circulations, distribution is described as the percentage of combined ventricular output, or CVO, the combined output of the left and right ventricles.

The percentage of CVO in various areas of the heart and other vessels is shown in Figure 4–5.[28] For obvious reasons, little of this information is available from human fetuses at term; the values depicted in the figure were obtained from unanesthetized chronically catheterized term sheep fetuses.

The sheep fetus at term is the same weight as the human fetus (approximately 3 kg), but species differences may occur (e.g., in the proportion of blood flow to the brain). Values of blood flow in milliliters per kilogram of fetal body weight per minute are shown in Figure 4–6. It should be noted that

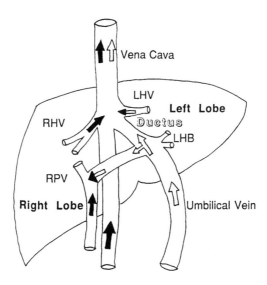

**FIGURE 4–2.** Ductus venosus. Diagram of the umbilical and hepatic circulations. Open arrows represent well-oxygenated blood, while the closed arrows represent less-oxygenated blood. RPV, right portal vein; RHV, right hepatic vein; LHV, left hepatic vein; LHB, left hepatic branch; Ductus, ductus venosus. (From Arnold-Aldea SA, Parer JT. Fetal cardiovascular physiology. In Eden RD, Boehm FH, Haire M, eds. Assessment and Care of the Fetus. Appleton & Lange, Norwalk, CT, 1990. Used by permission).

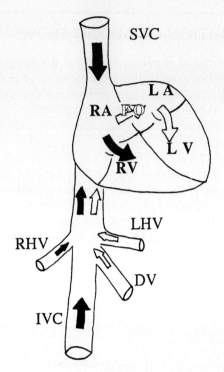

**FIGURE 4–3.** Blood flow through the inferior vena cava and foramen ovale. Open arrows represent well-oxygenated blood, while the closed arrows represent less-oxygenated blood. Well-oxygenated blood preferentially flows across the foramen ovale into the left atrium, while less-oxygenated blood flows into the right atrium. IVC, inferior vena cava; DV, ductus venosus; LHV, left hepatic vein; RHV, right hepatic vein; RA, right atrium; FO, foramen ovale; LA, left atrium; RV, right ventricle; LV, left ventricle; SVC, superior vena cava. (From Arnold-Aldea SA, Parer JT. Fetal cardiovascular physiology. In Eden RD, Boehm FH, Haire M, eds. Assessment and Care of the Fetus. Appleton & Lange, Norwalk, CT, 1990. Used by permission).

the combined ventricular output is 450 ml · $kg^{-1}$ · $min^{-1}$, with twice the quantity from the right as from the left ventricle. Approximately 45 percent of the CVO is umbilical blood flow (i.e., approximately 200 ml · $kg^{-1}$ · $min^{-1}$).

The estimated cardiac output of the human fetus (553 ml · $kg^{-1}$ · $min^{-1}$) is higher than that of the sheep (450 ml · $kg^{-1}$ · $min^{-1}$). In addition, the right and left ventricular outputs are more similar in the human compared to the sheep.[9] The ratio of right to left ventricular outputs decreases with advancing gestation, from 1.3 at 15 weeks to 1.1 at 40 weeks. These data are consistent with the fact that the larger human fetal brain requires a higher left ventricular output than the brain of the sheep.

Distribution of the cardiac output occurs in proportion to the vascular resistance of each bed. The percentage distributions of the cardiac output in normoxic fetal sheep are shown in Table 4–1. Note that the major part of the CVO perfuses the umbilical and carcass areas. The vascular resistances of each region are markedly changed during asphyxia, giving rise to preferential blood flow to certain vital organs (see later).

## III  FETAL BLOOD PRESSURES

The fetus is surrounded by a fluid-filled amniotic cavity, so fetal blood pressures must be related to the pressure of amniotic fluid. In the absence of uterine contractions, this pressure is generally stable.

The systemic arterial blood pressure of the fetus is considerably lower than that of the adult, averaging 55 mm Hg (systolic/diastolic, approximately 70/45 mm Hg) at term. Right ventricular pressure, 70/4 mm Hg, is slightly

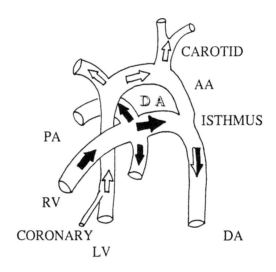

**FIGURE 4–4.**   The course of blood flow from the ventricles into the aorta. The ductus arteriosus allows the right and left ventricles to jointly perfuse the lower body. The upper body is perfused by well-oxygenated blood from the left ventricle. Open arrows represent well-oxygenated blood, while the closed arrows represent less-oxygenated blood. LV, left ventricle; RV, right ventricle; PA, pulmonary artery; DA, ductus arteriosus; AA, ascending aorta; DA, descending aorta. (From Arnold-Aldea SA, Parer JT. Fetal cardiovascular physiology. In Eden RD, Boehm FH, Haire M, eds. Assessment and Care of the Fetus. Appleton & Lange, Norwalk, CT, 1990. Used by permission).

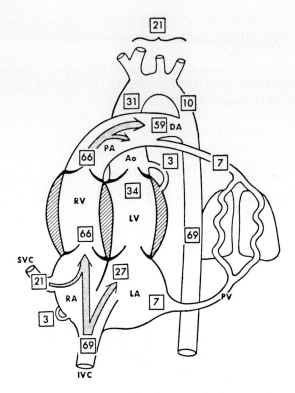

**FIGURE 4–5.** The distribution of blood flow in the heart and major vessels of a fetal sheep. Numbers represent the percentage of combined ventricular output in various areas. (From Rudolph AM. Congenital Diseases of the Heart. Year Book Medical Publishers, Chicago, 1974. Used by permission.)

greater (1 to 2 mm Hg) than left ventricular pressure. Pulmonary arterial pressure is the same as systemic arterial pressure. There is a slightly greater pressure in the right atrium (3 mm Hg) than in the left atrium (2 mm Hg), thus ensuring right-to-left blood flow across the foramen ovale.

Systemic blood pressures are somewhat lower earlier in gestation. This difference is reflected in the fact that premature newborns have a lower blood pressure than do term infants. Thus, at 30 weeks of gestation, the mean arterial blood pressure is only 35 mm Hg.

## IV  FACTORS CONTROLLING FETAL HEART RATE

Fetal heart rate (FHR) analysis is the prime means by which a fetus is evaluated for adequacy of oxygenation, so knowledge of its rate and regulation are of great importance to the obstetrician.

The average heart rate in the normal term fetus before labor is 140 beats/min. Earlier in pregnancy it is higher than this, although not substantially so. At 20 weeks the average FHR is 155 beats/min, and at 30 weeks of pregnancy it is 144 beats/min. Variations of 20 beats/min above or below these values are seen in normal fetuses.

The fetal heart is similar to that of the adult, in that it has its own intrinsic pacemaker activity that results in rhythmic contractions. The sinoatrial (SA) node, which is found in one wall of the right atrium, has the fastest rate of contraction and sets the rate in the normal heart (Fig. 4–7). The next fastest pacemaker rate is found in the atrium. Finally, the ventricle has a slower rate of beating than either the SA node or the atrium. In cases of complete or partial heart block in the fetus, variations in rate below normal can be seen. Typically, a fetus with a complete heart block has a rate of about 50 to 60 beats/min.

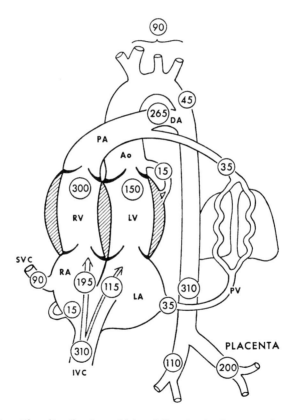

**FIGURE 4–6.** The distribution of blood flow in the heart and major vessels of the fetal sheep. Numbers represent the blood flow, in milliliters per kilogram of the fetus per minute, in various areas. (From Rudolph AM. Congenital Diseases of the Heart. Year Book Medical Publisher, Chicago, 1974. Used by permission.)

**TABLE 4–1.  Cardiac Output and Its Percentage Distribution in the Normoxic Fetal Lamb**

| | |
|---|---|
| Cardiac output | $450 \text{ ml} \cdot \text{kg}^{-1} \cdot \text{min}^{-1}$ |
| Placental blood flow | 40% |
| Lungs | 9% |
| Gastrointestinal tract | 5% |
| Brain | 4% |
| Myocardium | 3% |
| Kidneys | 3% |
| Spleen | 1% |
| Liver | 0.3% |
| Adrenal glands | 0.1% |
| Carcass (musculoskeletal system and skin) | 35% |

Variability of the FHR from beat to beat, and longer-term trends in heart rate over periods of less than a minute, are important properties. Variability is of great prognostic importance clinically; valuable empiric interpretations can be made from its presence and also from its decrease or absence.

The mean fetal heart rate is the result of many physiologic factors that modulate the intrinsic rate of the heart, the most obvious being signals from the autonomic nervous system.

# A  Parasympathetic Nervous System

The parasympathetic nervous system consists primarily of the vagus nerve (10th cranial nerve), which originates in the medulla oblongata. Fibers from this nerve supply the SA node and also the atrioventricular (AV) node, the neuronal bridge between atrium and ventricle (Fig. 4–7). Stimulation of the vagus nerve or injection of acetylcholine, the substance secreted at the nerve endings, results in a decrease in heart rate in the normal fetus owing to vagal influence on the SA node that decreases its rate of firing and the rate of transmission of impulses from atrium to ventricle. In a similar fashion, blocking of this nerve in a normal fetus by injecting a substance that blocks the effect of acetylcholine (e.g., atropine) causes an increase in the FHR of approximately 20 beats/min at term.[22] This finding demonstrates that there is normally a constant vagal influence on the FHR tending to decrease it from its normal intrinsic rate.

The vagus nerve apparently also has another very important function: it is responsible for transmission of impulses causing beat-to-beat variability of FHR. Blocking the vagus nerve with atropine results in a disappearance of this variability. Hence, it has been postulated that there are two vagal influences on the heart, the first, a tonic influence tending to decrease its rate, and the second, an oscillatory influence that results in FHR variability.[8] The vagal tone is not necessarily constant. Its influence increases with gestational age.[30] In fetal sheep vagal activity increases as much as fourfold during acute hypoxia[25] or experimentally produced fetal growth retardation.[19]

## **B** Sympathetic Nervous System

Sympathetic nerves are widely distributed in the muscle of the heart at term (Fig. 4–7). Stimulation of the sympathetic nerves will release norepinephrine

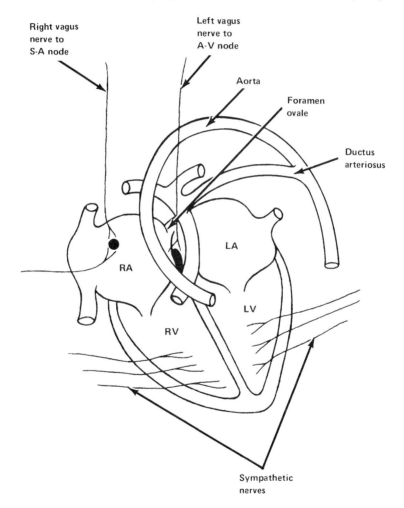

**FIGURE 4–7.** The fetal heart and its nervous connections. RA and LA, right and left atria; RV and LV, right and left ventricle. (From Parer JT. Physiological regulation of fetal heart rate. J Obstet Gynecol Neonatal Nurs 1976; 5:265–295. Used by permission.)

and cause increases in FHR and the vigor of cardiac contractions, resulting in higher cardiac output. The sympathetic nerves are a reserve mechanism to improve the pumping activity of the heart during intermittent stressful situations. There is normally a tonic sympathetic influence on the heart. Propranolol, which blocks the action of these sympathetic nerves, causes a decrease in FHR of approximately 10 beats/min when administered to the normal sheep fetus. As with the vagal tone, tonic influence increases as much as twofold during fetal hypoxia.

Fetal heart rate variability decreases only slightly after blocking of the sympathetic nerves in primates. There is a commonly held theory that FHR variability is a result of the two neuronal inputs to the fetal heart, vagal and beta-adrenergic, each with a different time constant. Because atropine almost abolishes FHR variability, and propranolol decreases it only a little, it is very unlikely that the theory is correct for the primate.[26] However, there may be an important species difference in the transmission of FHR variability impulses. Both vagal and beta-adrenergic influences are probably important in the sheep.[6] One must keep this in mind, because sheep are used so frequently in fetal physiology studies.

Alpha-adrenergic activity is also important in altering the distribution of blood flow to specific organs during stress. Thus, during hypoxia there is vasoconstriction of certain vascular beds (e.g., gut, liver, lung) that allows preferential flow of blood with the available oxygen to vital organs (e.g., brain, heart, and adrenals), and blood flow to the placenta is maintained (see later).

Several factors cause the parasympathetic and sympathetic nervous systems to increase their activity; they are discussed in the following pages.

## C  Chemoreceptors

Chemoreceptors are found both in the peripheral and in the central nervous systems. They have their most dramatic effects on the regulation of respiration, but they are still important in the control of the circulation. The peripheral chemoreceptors are in the carotid and aortic bodies, which are found in the arch of the aorta and the area of the carotid sinus (Fig. 4–8). The central chemoreceptors are in the medulla oblongata and respond to changes in the oxygen and carbon dioxide tensions in blood or cerebrospinal fluid perfusing this area.

In the adult, when oxygen in the arterial blood perfusing the central chemoreceptors is decreased or the carbon dioxide content is increased, a reflex tachycardia ordinarily develops. There is also a very substantial increase in arterial blood pressure, particularly with increases in carbon dioxide concentration; both of these effects are thought to be protective, in an attempt to circulate more blood through the affected areas in order to bring about a

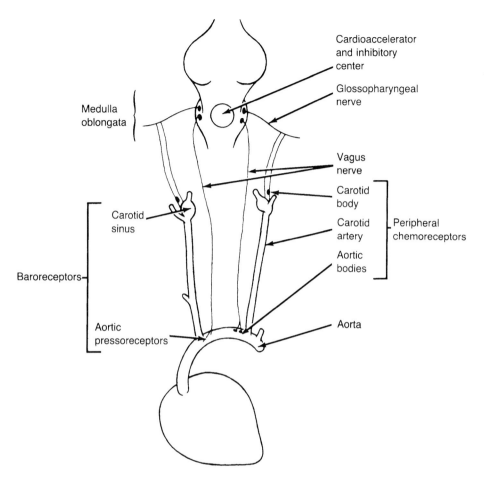

**FIGURE 4–8.** The peripheral chemo- and baroreceptors and their input to the cardiac integrating center in the medulla oblongata. (From Parer JT. Physiologic regulation of fetal heart rate. J Obstet Gynecol Neonatal Nurs 1976; 5:265–295. Used by permission.)

decrease in carbon dioxide tension or an increase in oxygen tension. Selective hypoxia or hypercapnia of the peripheral chemoreceptors alone in the adult produces a bradycardia, in contrast to the tachycardia and hypertension seen with central hypoxia or hypercapnia.

The interaction of the central and peripheral chemoreceptors in the fetus is poorly understood. It is known, however, that the net result of hypoxia or hypercapnia in the unanesthetized fetus is bradycardia with hypertension. During basal conditions, they seem to contribute to stabilize heart rate and blood pressure.[14]

## D  Baroreceptors

In the arch of the aorta and in the carotid sinus at the junction of the internal and external carotid arteries are small stretch receptors in the vessel walls that are sensitive to increases in blood pressure (Fig. 4–8). When pressure rises, impulses are sent from these receptors via the vagus or glossopharyngeal nerve to the mid-brain, resulting in further impulses via the vagus nerve to the heart, tending to slow it. This is an extremely rapid response, being seen with almost the first systolic rise of blood pressure. It is a protective, stabilizing attempt by the body to lower blood pressure by decreasing heart rate and cardiac output when blood pressure is increasing.

## E  Central Nervous System

It has been established that in the adult the higher centers of the brain influence heart rate (Fig. 4–9). Heart rate is increased by various emotional

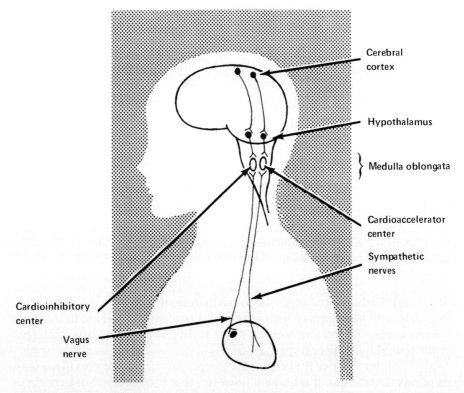

**FIGURE 4–9.** Schematic depiction of regulation of heart rate from the higher centers. (From Parer JT. Physiological regulation of fetal heart rate. J Obstet Gynecol Neonatal Nurs 1976; 5:265–295. Used by permission.)

stimuli, such as fear and sexual arousal. In fetal lambs and monkeys, the electroencephalogram or electrooculogram shows increased activity at times in association with variability of the heart rate and body movements. At other times, apparently when the fetus is sleeping, body movement slows and the FHR variability decreases, suggesting an association between these two factors and central nervous system activity.

The hypothalamus is thought to be the area of dispatch of nerve impulses produced by physical expressions of emotion, including acceleration of the heart rate and elevation of the blood pressure. It has been shown in the fetal lamb that stimulating an electrode in the hypothalamus causes the FHR to increase, at least initially, followed by a decrease, probably because of the protective baroreflex mentioned earlier. The increases in blood pressure and heart rate appear to be mediated by the sympathetic nerves.

The medulla oblongata contains the vasomotor centers, integrative centers where the net result of all the inputs is either acceleration or deceleration of the heart rate. This center is probably also where the net result of numerous central and peripheral inputs is processed to generate irregular oscillatory vagal impulses, giving rise to FHR variability.

## F  Hormonal Regulation

### ADRENAL MEDULLA
The fetal adrenal medulla produces epinephrine and norepinephrine in response to stressful situations (e.g., asphyxia). Both of these substances act on the heart and cardiovascular system in a way similar to sympathetic stimulation; that is, they produce a faster heart rate, greater force of contraction of the heart, and higher arterial blood pressure. However, it is not clear whether catecholamines exert a regulatory function in the resting fetus, at least in sheep.

### RENIN-ANGIOTENSIN SYSTEM
Angiotensin II seems to play a role in fetal circulatory regulation at rest, but its main activity is observed during hemorrhagic stress on a fetus.

### ARGININE VASOPRESSIN
Vasopressin has been shown to affect the distribution of blood flow in fetal sheep. However, this is presumably operative during hypoxia and possibly other stressful situations. A possible influence of arginine vasopressin on producing the sinusoidal FHR pattern is discussed in Chapter 9.

### PROSTAGLANDINS
Arachidonic acid metabolites are found in high concentrations in the fetal circulation and in many tissues. Their main role seems to be in the regulation

of umbilical blood flow as well as in maintaining the patency of the ductus arteriosus during fetal life.

## OTHER HUMORAL FACTORS

Other humoral factors such as nitric oxide, α-melanocyte-stimulating hormone (α-MSH), atrial natriuretic hormone, neuropeptide Y, thyrotropin-releasing hormone (TRH), and metabolites such as adenosine have also been described to be present in the fetus and to participate in the regulation of the fetal circulation.

# G Blood Volume Control

## CAPILLARY FLUID SHIFT

In the adult, when the blood pressure of the body is elevated by excessive blood volume, some fluid moves out of the capillaries into interstitial spaces, thereby decreasing the blood volume toward normal. Conversely, if the adult loses blood through hemorrhage, some fluid shifts out of the interstitial spaces into the circulation, thereby increasing the blood volume toward normal. There is normally a delicate balance between the pressures inside and outside the capillaries. This mechanism to regulate blood pressure is slower than the almost-instantaneous regulation found with the reflex mechanisms discussed previously. Its role in the fetus is imperfectly understood, although imbalances may be responsible for the hydrops seen in some cases of Rh isoimmunization and extreme fetal tachycardia. In addition, studies performed on sheep show that a fetus appears to be able to keep its blood volume closer to normal than an adult after reductions or expansions of volume.[3]

## INTRAPLACENTAL PRESSURES

Fluid moves down hydrostatic pressure gradients and also in response to osmotic pressure gradients. The actual value of these factors within the human placenta, where fetal and maternal blood closely approximate, is controversial. It seems likely, however, that there are some delicate balancing mechanisms within the placenta that prevent rapid fluid shifts between mother and fetus. The arterial blood pressure of the mother is much higher (approximately 100 mmHg) than that of the fetus (approximately 55 mmHg), and osmotic pressures are not substantially different. Hence, some compensatory mechanism must be present to equalize the effective pressures at the exchange points.

One such possibility is the existence of transtrophoblastic channels whose dimensions increase in response to an increase in fetal venous pressure, thus allowing intraplacental water passage. On return to normal fetal venous pressure, the channels disappear. Such channels for water may also allow transport of water-soluble, lipid-insoluble molecules.[17]

# H Cardiac Output Regulation

The amount of blood pumped by the heart is determined by the amount of blood returning to the heart; that is, the heart pumps all of the blood that flows into it without excessive damming of blood in the veins. When the cardiac muscle is stretched prior to contraction by an increased inflow of blood, it contracts with a greater force than before and is able to pump out more blood. This mechanism, known as the Frank–Starling mechanism, has been studied in the unanesthetized fetal lamb and has been shown to be less well developed than in the adult sheep,[29] probably because the fetal heart muscle is not as well developed. It is likely that the same is true of the human fetus, which is generally more immature at birth than the lamb. As a consequence, increases in the filling pressure or preload produce minor if any changes in combined ventricular output, suggesting that the fetal heart normally operates near the top of its function curve.

The output of the fetal heart is also related to the heart rate. Some investigators have shown that spontaneous variations of heart rate relate directly to cardiac output; that is, as rate increases, output increases. However, different responses have been observed during right or left atrial pacing studies. No changes were observed in left ventricular output when the right atrium was paced, whereas the output decreased during left atrial pacing.[1] Similarly, right ventricular output was unchanged with left atrial pacing, and reduced with right atrial pacing.[2] Clearly, additional factors are operating to explain such differences. In addition to heart rate and preload, cardiac output depends on afterload and intrinsic contractility.[1, 2]

This relationship between FHR and cardiac output has not been confirmed in human fetuses under physiologic conditions, because the spontaneous increase in heart rate has been found to be associated with a decrease in stroke volume, maintaining the cardiac output unchanged.[18]

The fetal heart appears to be very sensitive to changes in the afterload, represented by the fetal arterial blood pressure. In this way, increases in afterload dramatically reduce the stroke volume or cardiac output. As has already been stated, the fetal heart is incompletely developed compared to that of adults. Many ultrastructural differences between the fetal and adult heart account for a lower intrinsic capacity of the fetal heart to contract. Each of these four determinants of cardiac output do not work separately, but rather they interact dynamically to modulate the fetal cardiac output during physiologic conditions. Cardiac output responses during hypoxic bradycardia are described later.

In clinical practice it is reasonable to assume that at modest variations of heart rate from the normal range, there are relatively small effects on the cardiac output. However, at extremes (e.g., a tachycardia above 240 or a bradycardia below 60 beats/min) cardiac output and umbilical blood flow are likely to be substantially decreased.

## V    UMBILICAL BLOOD FLOW

The umbilical blood flow in the undisturbed human at term is about 120 ml/kg/min, or 360 ml/min. Such measurements have been obtained by noninvasive methods using ultrasound techniques.[12, 13] This is somewhat higher than values obtained immediately after birth, but the latter are probably affected by cord manipulation during the birth process. The measurements have not yet found clinical applicability, but the same Doppler technique can be used to calculate the peak systolic:diastolic flow ratio, which is a reflection of vascular impedance distal to the point of measurement (see below).

The umbilical blood flow in the human is considerably less than that of the sheep, where it is approximately 200 ml $\cdot$ kg$^{-1}$ $\cdot$ min$^{-1}$.[15] The differences may be explained by the somewhat higher metabolic rate of the sheep (body temperature 39°C) and differences in hemoglobin concentrations (sheep, 10 g $\cdot$ dl$^{-1}$ versus human, 15 g $\cdot$ dl$^{-1}$). It is important to recognize this species difference because the bulk of our information regarding fetal circulatory physiology comes from the chronically instrumented sheep fetus. In sheep, the umbilical blood flow is approximately 45 percent of the combined ventricular output[15] and about 20 percent of this blood flow is "shunted," that is, it does not exchange with maternal blood. It is either carried through actual vascular shunts within the fetal side of the placenta or else it does not approach closely enough to maternal blood for exchange with it.

Umbilical blood flow is unaffected by acute moderate hypoxia but is decreased by severe hypoxia.[5] Innervation of the umbilical cord is questionable, but umbilical blood flow decreases with the administration of catecholamines. It is also decreased by acute cord occlusion. There are no known means of increasing umbilical flow in cases where it is thought to be decreased chronically. However, certain FHR patterns (i.e., variable decelerations) have been ascribed to transient umbilical cord compression in the fetus during labor. Manipulation of maternal position either to the lateral or Trendelenburg position can sometimes abolish these patterns, the implication being that cord compression has been relieved.

## VI    DOPPLER VELOCIMETRY

### A    Blood Velocity Waveforms

Real-time directed Doppler ultrasound has been used to investigate human fetal, placental, and uterine blood flows.[31] Doppler ultrasound allows measurement of velocity waveforms of red cells traveling in vessels. The velocity data can be used to make inferences about blood flow, vascular resistance, and myocardial contractility. Blood flow velocity waveforms have a characteristic appearance that varies from vessel to vessel. The observed waveform shape is affected by the pumping ability of the heart, the heart rate, the elasticity of the vessel wall, the outflow impedance, and the blood viscosity. Waveforms in arteries supplying low-resistance vascular beds have a characteristically high forward velocity during diastole, while absent or reverse diastolic flow is seen in arteries supplying high-resistance vascular beds. These observations prompted the definition of indices of flow that could be related to the vascular resistance of a downstream vascular bed. The most commonly used indices are:

$$\text{Pulsatility index: PI} = V_{max} - V_{min}/V_{mean}$$
$$\text{Pourcelot ratio: PR} = V_{max} - V_{min}/V_{max}$$
$$\text{AB(SD) ratio: AB} = V_{max}/V_{min}$$

where

$V_{max}$ = point of maximal blood flow velocity per cardiac cycle
$V_{min}$ = point of minimal blood flow velocity per cardiac cycle
$V_{mean}$ = mean blood flow velocity per cardiac cycle

In normal pregnancy, high forward velocity levels in the umbilical artery are maintained throughout diastole. A lowered diastolic flow, as seen in severe intrauterine growth retardation, may reflect raised placental resistance.[11] Clinical aspects of Doppler velocimetry are discussed in Chapter 2.

## B  Volume Blood Flow

Doppler ultrasound permits estimation of blood flows in the human fetus. Blood flow (Q) is calculated using the formula:

$$Q = (V \times A)/\text{Cos } \theta$$

where

$V$ = mean velocity as averaged over many cardiac cycles (cm • sec$^{-1}$)
$A$ = estimated cross-sectional area of the vessel (cm$^2$)
$\theta$ = angle between the Doppler beam and the direction of flow of the blood

This calculation is complicated by the variation in the velocity of blood cells across a vascular lumen. Cells flow faster in the center of the vessel and slower near the vessel wall. The overall flow in a vessel is the sum of the different flows across the lumen. For this reason, satisfactory volume flow measurements can best be made on large vessels (4 to 10 mm in diameter) with appropriate Doppler angles (30 to 60 degrees).[12, 13]

The two-dimensional echo Doppler provides a means of estimating fetal cardiac output by quantifying blood flow volume at the AV valve orifices. As noted previously, the estimated cardiac output of the human fetus (553 ml $\cdot$ kg$^{-1}$ $\cdot$ min$^{-1}$) is higher than that of the sheep (450 ml $\cdot$ kg$^{-1}$ $\cdot$ min$^{-1}$). In addition, the right and left ventricular outputs are more similar in the human compared to the sheep. The ratio of right to left ventricular outputs decreases with advancing gestation, from 1.3 at 15 weeks to 1.1 at 40 weeks. These data are consistent with the fact that the larger human brain requires a higher left ventricular output than the brain of the sheep.

These estimates of the volume of blood flow require considerable expertise and time to obtain accurate results, and at present are of research rather than clinical value.

# VII HYPOXIA/ASPHYXIA

## A Fetal Responses

Studies of chronically prepared animals have shown that a number of responses occur during acute hypoxia or asphyxia in the previously normoxic fetus. There is little or no change in combined cardiac output and umbilical (placental) blood flow, but there is a redistribution of blood flow favoring certain vital organs—namely, heart, brain, and adrenal glands—and a decrease in the blood flow to the gut, spleen, kidneys, and carcass[4] (Fig. 4–10). This initial response is presumed to be advantageous to a fetus in the same way as the diving reflex is in an adult seal, in that the blood containing the available oxygen and other nutrients is supplied preferentially to vital organs.

Fetal oxygen consumption decreased to values as low as 60 percent of control (from approximately 8 to 5 ml $\cdot$ kg$^{-1}$ $\cdot$ min$^{-1}$) during fetal hypoxia in the chronically instrumented fetus with arterial oxygen tension of 10 mmHg.[24] This decrease is rapidly instituted, stable for periods up to 45 minutes, proportional to the degree of hypoxia, and rapidly reversible on cessation of maternal hypoxia. It is accompanied by a fetal bradycardia of about 30 beats/min below control (approximately 170 beats/min control to 140 beats/min hypoxia in fetal sheep) and an increase in fetal arterial blood pressure (approximately 54 mmHg control to 61 mmHg hypoxia mean pressure). There is also progressive fetal acidosis during fetal isocapnic hypoxia (fetal arterial pH 7.38 control to 7.33 after 25 minutes hypoxia). This is a metabolic acidosis due to lactic acid accumulation as a result of anaerobic metabolism primarily in those partially vasoconstricted beds where oxygenation is inadequate for normal basic needs.[21] During fetal asphyxia, the increase in carbon dioxide tension superimposes a respiratory component on the acidosis.

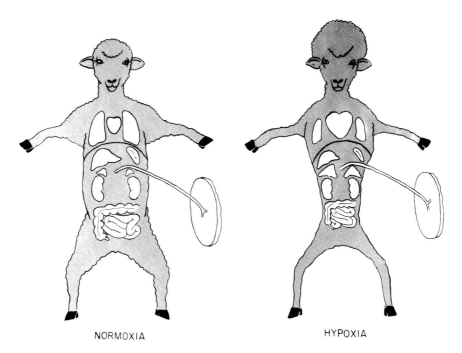

NORMOXIA                HYPOXIA

**FIGURE 4–10.**   A schematic illustration of the redistribution of blood flow that occurs during fetal hypoxia. The size of the organs and other regions of the fetus are in proportion to the quantity of blood flow. The head, heart, and adrenal glands are larger, and the placental size remains unchanged. Other organs and the body are smaller. (Courtesy of Dr. M. Lynne Reuss.)

The series of responses just described—that is, redistribution of blood flow favoring vital organs, decreased total oxygen consumption, and anaerobic glycolysis—may be thought of as temporary compensatory mechanisms that enable a fetus to survive moderately long periods (e.g., up to 30 minutes) of limited oxygen supply without decompensation of vital organs, particularly the brain and heart. The close matching of blood flow to oxygen availability to achieve a constancy of oxygen consumption has been demonstrated in the fetal cerebral circulation[16] and in the fetal myocardium.[10] In studies on hypoxic lamb fetuses, cerebral oxygen consumption was constant over a wide range of arterial oxygen contents because the decrease in arteriovenous oxygen content accompanying hypoxia was compensated for by an increase in cerebral blood flow.

However, during more severe asphyxia or sustained hypoxemia, these responses are no longer maintained, and a decrease in the cardiac output, arterial blood pressure, and blood flow to the brain and heart have been

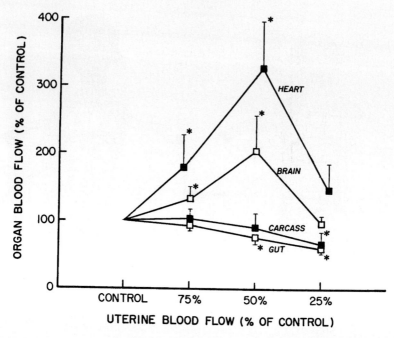

**FIGURE 4–11.** The effect of graded reductions in uterine blood flow on blood flow redistribution in the sheep fetus. When uterine blood flow is reduced to 75 percent of control, blood flow is preferentially redistributed to the heart and brain at the expense of other tissues or organs (e.g., carcass and gut). This redistribution is more pronounced when uterine blood flow is reduced to 50 percent of control value. However, when further reduced to 25 percent of control, the resultant severe asphyxia results in a partial "breakdown" of the blood flow redistribution mechanism. It is suggested that this leads to a reduction of myocardial and/or cerebral oxygen consumption (see text). (Modified from Yaffe H, Parer JT, Block BS, Llanos AJ. Cardiorespiratory responses to graded reductions of uterine blood flow in the sheep fetus. J Dev Physiol 1987; 9:325–336. Used by permission.)

described[32] (Fig. 4–11). These changes may be considered to be a stage of decompensation, after which tissue damage and even fetal death may follow[23] (see also Chapter 10).

## B  Metabolic Effects

It is known that the fetus depends partially on anaerobic metabolism for its energy needs during oxygen insufficiency.[20] It has also been shown in experimental animals that a newborn's ability to tolerate asphyxia depends on cardiac carbohydrate reserves. Whether this also applies to a human fetus is unknown, but clinical observations support the view that carbohydrate-depleted fetuses succumb more readily than those with normal reserves. A nutritionally growth-retarded fetus also is more susceptible to intrauterine asphyxia and depression than a normal fetus.

It has been stated that the prime aim of compensatory responses in hypoxia is maintenance of the circulation, and maintenance of the integrity of cardiac function is paramount in this regard. It is likely that carbohydrate availability is critical in supplying substrates for glycolysis at more severe degrees of hypoxia.

## C  Mechanisms of Responses

The cardiovascular responses to hypoxia are instituted rapidly and are mediated by neural and humoral mechanisms (Fig. 4–12). As has been previously mentioned, the tonic influence of the autonomic nervous system on heart rate, blood pressure, and the umbilical circulation in a normoxic fetus is quantitatively minor. This is in marked contrast to autonomic activity during hypoxia.

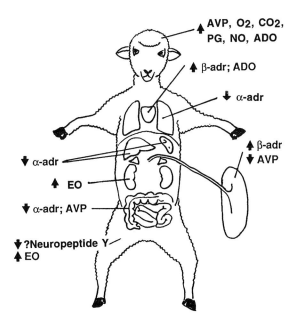

**FIGURE 4–12.**  Summary of the mechanisms that are known to participate in the regulation of blood flow due to changes in vascular resistance in different organs and tissues during hypoxia in the fetal sheep. ↑, increase in blood flow; ↓, decrease in blood flow. ADO, adenosine; *adr*, adrenergic; AVP, arginine vasopressin; EO, endogenous opioids; NO, nitric oxide, PG, prostaglandins.

In studies using total pharmacologic blockade, it has been shown that parasympathetic activity is augmented three to five times and β-adrenergic activity doubles when measured by heart rate response. The net result of these changes is a decrease in FHR during hypoxia.[5] Augmented β-adrenergic activity also may be important in maintaining cardiac output and umbilical blood flow during hypoxia, probably by increased inotropic effect on the heart.

Alpha-adrenergic activity is important in determining regional distribution of blood flow in hypoxic fetal sheep by selective vasoconstriction. As noted earlier, during hypoxia there is preferential blood flow to the brain, heart, and adrenals and decreased supply to the carcass, lungs, kidneys, and gut. Alpha-adrenergic blockade reversed the hypertension and increased peripheral resistance observed during fetal hypoxia. These changes are due to a decrease in the resistance in the gut, spleen, lungs, and probably carcass, indicating a participation of the α-adrenergic system in their vasoconstriction.[27]

Plasma concentrations of catecholamines, arginine vasopressin, β-endorphin, and atrial natriuretic factor increase during hypoxia in the fetus. The contributions of catecholamines to the circulatory responses to hypoxia have been described. Vasopressin contributes to the increase in blood pressure observed during hypoxia by decreasing umbilical and gut blood flows. Beta-endorphin and probably other endogenous opioids also participate in the response to hypoxia. The blockade of its receptors with naloxone further increases the hypertensive response by increasing the vasoconstriction in the kidneys and carcass. During hypoxia, a decrease in the fetal blood volume has been described. Atrial natriuretic factor may play a role in this response. In addition, nitric oxide, prostaglandins and adenosine have all been implicated in regulation of the fetal circulation during hypoxia (see Chapter 5).

Most of these results have been obtained from the chronically catheterized fetal sheep model. The relative contribution of these and other mediators to the cardiovascular response to hypoxia in a human fetus continue to be explored, because it is clear that the redistribution of blood flow is a powerful mechanism for protection of fetal organs from asphyxial damage during periods of oxygen insufficiency.

## REFERENCES

1. Anderson PAW, Glick KL, Killam AP, Mainwaring RD. The effect of heart rate on in utero left ventricular output in the fetal sheep. J Physiol 1986; 372:557–573.
2. Anderson PAW, Killam AP, Mainwaring RD, Oakeley AE. In utero right ventricular output in the fetal lamb: the effect of heart rate. J Physiol 1987; 387:297–316.

3. Brace RA. Current topic: Progress toward understanding the regulation of amniotic fluid volume: water and solute fluxes in and through the fetal membranes. Placenta 1995; 16:1–18.

4. Cohn HE, Sacks EJ, Heymann MA, Rudolph AM. Cardiovascular responses to hypoxemia and acidemia in fetal lambs. Am J Obstet Gynecol 1974; 120:817–824.

5. Court DJ, Parer JT. Experimental studies in fetal asphyxia and fetal heart rate interpretation. In Nathanielsz PW, Parer JT, eds. Research in Perinatal Medicine, Vol. 1. Perinatology Press, Ithaca, NY, 1985, pp. 114–164.

6. Dalton KJ, Phill D, Dawes GS, Patrick JE. The autonomic nervous system and fetal heart rate variability. Am J Obstet Gynecol 1983; 146:456–462.

7. Dawes GS. Fetal and Neonatal Physiology. Year Book Medical Publishers, Chicago, 1968.

8. De Hann J, Solte LAM, Veth AFL, et al. Die Bedeuting der schnellen Oszillationen im Kardiotachogramm des Feten. In Saling E, Dudenhausen JW, eds. Perinatale Medizin, Band III. Thieme, Stuttgart, 1972, 398.

9. De Smedt MC, Visser GH, Meijboom EJ. Fetal cardiac output estimated by Doppler echocardiography during mid- and late gestation. Am J Cardiol 1987; 60:338.

10. Fisher DJ, Heymann MA, Rudolph MA. Fetal myocardial oxygen and carbohydrate consumption during acutely induced bypoxemia. Am J Physio 1982; 242:H657.

11. Fleischer A, Schulman H, Farmakides G, et al. Umbilical velocity wave ratios in intrauterine growth retardation. Am J Obstet Gynecol 1985; 151:502–505.

12. Gill RW. Pulsed Doppler with B-mode imaging for quantitative blood flow measurement. Ultrasound Med Biol 1979; 5:223–235.

13. Gill RW, Trudinger BJ, Garrett WJ, et al. Fetal umbilical venous flow measured in utero by pulsed Doppler and B-mode ultrasound. Am J Obstet Gynecol 1981; 139: 720–725.

14. Hanson MA. The importance of baro- and chemo-reflexes in the control of the fetal cardiovascular system. J Dev Physiol 1988; 10:491–511.

15. Heymann MA. Fetal cardiovascular physiology. In Creasy RK, Resnik R, eds. Maternal-Fetal Medicine: Principles and Practice, 3rd ed. WB Saunders, Philadelphia, 1994, pp. 276–287.

16. Jones MD, Sheldon RE, Peeters LL, et al. Fetal cerebral oxygen consumption at different levels of oxygenation. J Appl Physiol 1977; 43:1080–1084.

17. Kaufmann P, Burton G. Anatomy and genesis of the placenta. Chapter 8 in Knobil E, Neill JD, eds. The Physiology of Reproduction. Raven Press, New York, 1994, pp. 441–483.

18. Kenny J, Plappert T, Doubilet P, et al. Effects of heart rate on ventricular size, stroke volume, and output in the normal human fetus: A prospective Doppler echocardiographic study. Circulation 1987; 76:52–58.

19. Llanos AJ, Green JR, Creasy RK, Rudolph AM. Increased heart rate response to parasympathetic and beta-adrenergic blockade in growth-retarded fetal lambs. Am J Obstet Gynecol 1980; 136:808–813.

20. Low JA, Pancham SR, Worthington D, Boston RW. The acid-base and biochemical characteristics of intrapartum fetal asphyxia. Am J Obstet Gynecol 1975; 121: 446–451.

21. Mann LI. Effects in sheep of hypoxia on levels of lactate, pyruvate, and glucose in blood of mothers and fetus. Pediatr Res 1970; 4:46–54.

22. Mendez-Bauer C, Poseirio JJ, Arellano-Hernandez G, et al. Effects of atropine on the heart rate of the human fetus during labor. Am J Obstet Gynecol 1963; 85:1033–1053.

23. Myers RE. Two patterns of brain damage and their conditions of occurrence. Am J Obstet Gynecol 1972; 112:246–276.

24. Parer JT. The effect of acute maternal hypoxia on fetal oxygenation and the umbilical circulation in the sheep. Eur J Obstet Gynecol Repro Biol 1980; 10:125–136.

25. Parer JT. The effect of atropine on heart rate and oxygen consumption of the hypoxic fetus. Am J Obstet Gynecol 1984; 148:1118–1122.

26. Parer JT, Laros RK, Keilbron DC, Krueger JR. The roles of parasympathetic and beta-adrenergic activity in beat-to-beat fetal heart rate variability. In Kovac AGB, Namos E, Rubanyi G, eds. Physiologic Science. Vol. 8: Cardiovascular Physiology. Pergamon Press, New York, 1981, pp. 327–330.

27. Reuss ML, Parer JT, Harris JL, Krueger TR. Hemodynamic effects of alpha-adrenergic blockade during hypoxia in fetal sheep. Am J Obstet Gynecol 1982; 142:410–415.

28. Rudolph AM. Congenital Diseases of the Heart. Year Book Medical Publishers, Chicago, 1974.

29. Rudolph AM, Heymann MA. Control of the foetal circulation. In Comline RS, Dawes GS, Nathanielsz PW, eds. Foetal and Neonatal Physiology: Proceedings, Sir Joseph Barcroft Centenary Symposium. Cambridge University Press, London, 1973.

30. Schifferli PY, Caldeyro-Barcia R. Effects of atropine and beta-adrenergic drugs on the heart rate of the human fetus. In Boreus, eds. Fetal Pharmacology. Raven Press, New York, 1973.

31. Trudinger BJ, Giles WB, Cook CM. Flow velocity wave-forms in the maternal uteroplacental and fetal placental circulation. Am J Obstet Gynecol 1985; 152:155–163.

32. Yaffe H, Parer JT, Block BS, Llanos AJ. Cardiorespiratory responses to graded reductions of uterine blood flow in the sheep fetus. J Dev Physiol 1987; 9:325–336.

# ■ *Chapter Five*

# Fetal Cerebral Metabolism

 FETAL BRAIN METABOLISM UNDER
CONDITIONS OF NORMAL OXYGENATION

## A Normal Values

### OXYGEN CONSUMPTION

Most measurements of fetal brain cerebral cortex oxygen consumption have been obtained in fetal sheep, with the modified Fick principle. Blood oxygen content is measured with catheters in the preductal (ascending) aorta and sagittal sinus, and cerebral cortical blood flow (CBF) is measured using the radionuclide microsphere technique. In the near-term fetal sheep the mean CBF is 120 ml • 100 $g^{-1}$ • $min^{-1}$, and arteriovenous oxygen content difference 1.6 mM. This results in a mean cerebral oxygen consumption rate of about 190 mM • 100 $g^{-1}$ • $min^{-1}$ (Table 5–1).[11]

The oxygen consumption is similar to this in the adult sheep and newborn.[12] However, in the fetus the oxygen delivery is 70 percent greater than that in the adult, implying an excessive blood flow for the resting needs (Fig. 5–1). Thus the fetal CBF is higher than that of the adult at any arterial oxygen content. This may be a physiologic adaptation to the lower partial pressure of oxygen in the fetal blood, or a reserve mechanism for anticipated stressful conditions.[9]

In adults and newborns it is estimated that approximately half of the oxygen consumption supplies energy for synaptic transmission. One quarter of the oxygen consumption maintains neuronal membrane potentials, and a further one quarter is devoted to unidentified processes.[12]

71

## TABLE 5–1.    Fetal Sheep Brain Metabolism

|  | Near Term | ~90 d |
|---|---|---|
| Oxygen consumption ($\mu M \cdot 100\ g^{-1} \cdot min^{-1}$) | 180 | 45 |
| Glucose consumption ($\mu M \cdot 100\ g^{-1} \cdot min^{-1}$) | 30 | 8.5 |
| Lactate production ($\mu mol \cdot 100\ g^{-1} \cdot min^{-1}$) | 0 | 2.5 |
| Cortical blood flow (ml $\cdot 100\ g^{-1} \cdot min^{-1}$) | 120 | 34 |

See Parer[16] for sources of data.

## CARBOHYDRATE METABOLISM

Glucose consumption in the near-term fetal sheep is approximately 26 mM $\cdot$ 100 $g^{-1} \cdot min^{-1}$ (Table 5–1). The oxygen–glucose index, which is a measure of the extent to which complete metabolism of the glucose can explain the total oxygen uptake, is 100 percent in such sheep, suggesting that glucose is the major and possibly only substrate used by the brain under

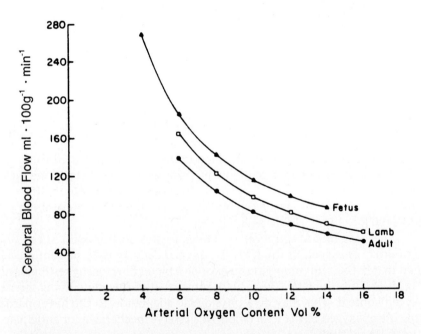

**FIGURE 5–1.**    The relationship between CBF and ascending aortic arterial blood oxygen content. Note that the fetus has a CBF over 50 percent greater than that of the adult. (From Jones MD Jr, Traystman RJ. Cerebral oxygenation of the fetus, newborn, and adult. Semin Perinatol 1984; 8:205–216. Reprinted with permission.)

normal conditions. However, recent work points to a portion of the energy during the low-voltage state (with higher metabolic rates) being supplied anaerobically from glucose.

## B   Developmental Changes

Oxygen consumption in fetal sheep at 93 days (0.63 gestation) is approximately 50 mM $\cdot$ 100 $g^{-1} \cdot min^{-1}$, that is 25 percent of the value in the near-term fetus.[6] This reduced metabolism occurs in the face of a reduced CBF rather than a reduction in fractional oxygen extraction or arteriovenous oxygen content difference across the brain (Table 5–1). This lower oxygen uptake may reflect less developed synaptic activity, and may also be a consequence of the lesser mitochondrial mass in the immature brain.[6]

In the sheep fetus at 0.63 of gestation the cerebral glucose consumption is 8.5 mM $\cdot$ 100 $g^{-1} \cdot min^{-1}$, that is, 30 percent of that in the near-term sheep fetus (Table 5–1). There is net lactate production under normal conditions, which can explain a further 15 percent of the glucose utilization, and together with the glucose, essentially all of the oxygen consumption. Because of the high oxygen values in fetal sheep blood there is no reason to believe lactate is a result of insufficient oxygen availability.[6]

## C   Influence of Fetal State

The fetal sheep near term spends the most time in the low-voltage state, during which time rapid eye and rapid irregular breathing movements occur. Measurements in chronically prepared fetal sheep show that during the high-voltage state the cerebral oxygen consumption is 83 percent of that found in the more active low-voltage state. The difference may represent increased brain neuronal activity, or an increase in synthesis within the brain in the low-voltage state.[19, 20]

As with oxygen consumption, the glucose consumption in the fetus is also increased during low-voltage electrocortical activity (see also the section on carbohydrate metabolism, above). Glucose consumption has been shown to be dependent on auditory input in the near-term fetal sheep. In fetuses with cochlear ablation, using the radioactive carbon ($^{14}$C) deoxyglucose method, local glucose utilization was depressed in most of the gray and white matter examined, and was reduced 25 percent in brain stem auditory nuclei. Furthermore, glucose utilization in many cerebral structures was elevated in noise exposed fetuses (reviewed by Parer[16]).

## D   Regulation of Fetal Brain Metabolism (Table 5–2)

In the adult brain there is acceptance of the concept that local CBF is normally distributed in almost the exact proportion to the rates of glucose utilization, and that the blood flow and local glucose consumption change in response to

**TABLE 5–2.   Regulation of Fetal Cortical Blood Flow During Normoxia**

Local CBF is closely coupled to rate of glucose utilization
Varies inversely with oxygen content
Varies directly with carbon dioxide tension
Humoral agents (e.g., nitric oxide)
Autoregulation
   Stable CBF over a range of perfusion pressures
   Narrower blood pressure range in preterm fetuses, and blood pressure is close
   to lower limit of autoregulation

local functional activity.[23] This coupling is relatively poorly studied in the sheep under "normal" conditions, but more is known under pathologic perturbations.

Variations in CBF can be due to variations in oxygen content and carbon dioxide levels of arterial blood. Even within the normal range blood flow increases as oxygen decreases, resulting in a constant cerebral oxygen consumption.[10, 11] Szymonowicz et al.,[24] however, concluded that CBF was not primarily determined by oxygen content when variations occurred within the physiologic range. In addition to oxygen control, it is known that CBF increases as carbon dioxide tension increases.[10, 18, 22] Nitric oxide may play a role in normal regulation as blockade causes an increase in cerebral vascular resistance in the normally oxygenated fetal lamb.[27]

Autoregulation of CBF occurs in the adult and also in the fetus.[15, 18, 26] Thus there is a range of arterial blood pressure over which CBF remains stable. It has been shown that in the preterm lamb the range is narrowed, compared to the term lamb, and that the mean resting carotid arterial blood pressure lies close to the lower limit of autoregulation[15] (Fig. 5–2).

---

## II   FETAL BRAIN METABOLISM DURING ASPHYXIA

## A   Fetal Cerebral Oxygen Consumption During Induced Hypoxia/Asphyxia

During hypoxia or asphyxia produced in the fetal sheep by various techniques, there is a decrease in cerebral vascular resistance and an increase in CBF.[4, 11, 17, 18] The increase in blood flow is such that the oxygen consumption of the cerebral hemispheres remains constant over the range of ascending aortic oxygen tensions of 14 to 36 mmHg.[11] Arterial oxygen content has the best overall correlation with CBF among different types of hypoxia.[12] In addition to the role of decreased oxygen in bringing about this vasodilitation, increasing carbon dioxide tension is also involved in vasodilation of the cerebral vascular bed during asphyxia.[18, 22]

In the mid-term fetal sheep there is an increase in CBF during hypoxia but this is less than that seen in the term fetus, so that oxygen consumption of the brain is maintained by combined increased fractional oxygen oxtraction and increased blood flow.[7] The authors suggested that this may have been due to immature regulatory mechanisms.

As noted above autoregulation has been demonstrated in the fetal lamb, such that blood flow to the brain is maintained nearly constant over a wide range of arterial pressures. This autoregulation has been shown to be dependent on an adequate level of arterial oxygen, because during hypoxia cerebral blood flow became pressure dependent[26] (Fig. 5–3).

Under conditions of severe asphyxia when uterine blood flow was 25 percent of control, it was found that sufficient augmentation of the cerebral blood flow was no longer maintained, and similar values to control were obtained (see Fig. 4–11). There was a doubling of the vascular resistance in the cerebral vasculature compared to normoxic control values, and a further

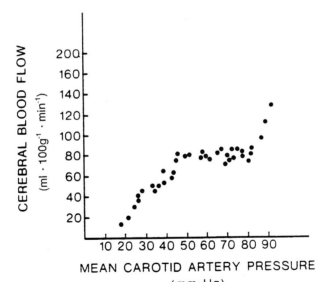

**FIGURE 5–2.**    Autoregulation of CBF in the premature (approx. 0.6 gestation) fetal lamb. Cerebral blood flow remains relatively constant over the arterial blood pressure range of 45 to 80 mmHg. Outside this range it is related to the arterial blood pressure. (From Papile L-A, Rudolph AM, Heyman MA. Autoregulation of cerebral blood flow in preterm fetal lamb. Pediatr Res 1985; 19:159–161. Reprinted with permission.)

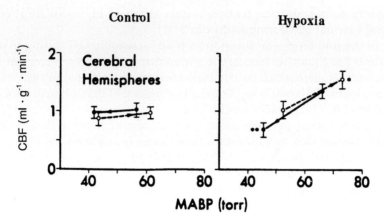

**FIGURE 5–3.**    Cerebral blood flow related to fetal mean arterial blood pressure. Under control conditions there is autoregulation with constancy of CBF at varying pressures. This constancy (or autoregulation) is lost under hypoxic conditions. Arrows show the direction of experimental change in pressure. (From Tweed WA, Cote J, Pash M, Lou H. Arterial oxygenation determines autoregulation of cerebral blood flow in the fetal lamb. Pediatr Res 1983; 17:246–249. Reprinted with permission.)

increase in arterial blood pressure. This decrease in blood flow, coupled with a decreased arteriovenous oxygen difference during more profound hypoxemia, results in a decrease in cerebral oxygen consumption to as much as half of normal.[5] This reduced consumption appears to be proportional to the degree of hypoxemia as measured by arterial oxygen content (Fig. 5–4), and is due to the fact that cerebral vascular resistance does not decrease further in response to and in proportion to the increasing hypoxemia. Thus CBF can no longer be augmented below a certain level of hypoxemia, and with the progressive obligatory reduction in arteriovenous oxygen difference, the uptake of oxygen falls. The reduction in cerebral oxygen consumption appears to occur when ascending aorta oxygen content is below 1 mM. A decrease in cerebral oxygen consumption was also demonstrated to occur after 7.2 hours of isocapnic hypoxia in fetal sheep when the arterial oxygen content was below 0.8 mM.[21]

The inability of the fetus to maintain sufficient oxygen delivery to the brain had previously been predicted in the basis of the increased fraction of cardiac output (from 25 to 50 percent) required to be directed toward the heart and central nervous system. On the basis of mathematical modeling it was suggested that when ascending aortic oxygen content was reduced from 1 to 0.5 mmol/$L^{-1}$ such a compensation could not take place, and the cardiovascular system may begin to fail in delivering adequate amounts of oxygen to at least some parts of the central nervous system.

## B Carbohydrate Metabolism During Asphyxia

During hypoxia/asphyxia of moderate to severe degrees the circulating glucose concentration rises by approximately 50 percent in fetal sheep. Similarly, there is development of a metabolic acidosis, most of which can be explained by increased lactate levels.[8]

The glucose and lactate flux across the brain has been studied in the fetal sheep during cerebral ischemia produced by partial occlusion of the brachiocephalic artery.[3] During severe ischemia there is reduced brain oxygen consumption, approximately 26 percent, and increased glucose uptake, approximately 25 percent (Fig. 5–5). This is considerably more glucose than can account for the oxygen uptake. The brain lost lactate during occlusion, but not to a degree sufficient to explain anaerobic metabolism of the glucose. The authors concluded that lactate accumulated in the brain tissue because of inability of the blood–brain barrier to transport it, and that this may contribute to brain injury, in which elevated lactate levels have been

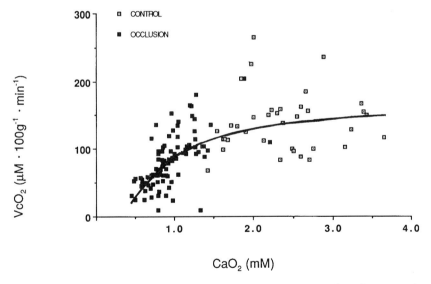

**FIGURE 5–4.** Fetal cerebral oxygen consumption (VcO$_2$) related to ascending aortic oxygen content (CaO$_2$). The open symbols are control values, and the solid symbols during asphyxia induced by temporary uterine artery occlusion. Note the tendency for V̇cO$_2$ to decline at CaO$_2$'s below 1 mM. (From Field DR, Parer JT, Auslender RA, et al. Cerebral oxygen consumption during asphyxia in fetal sheep. J Dev Physiol 1990; 14:131–137. Reprinted with permission.)

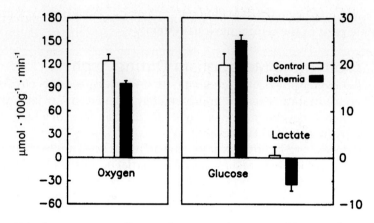

**FIGURE 5–5.** Net fluxes of oxygen, glucose, and lactate during experimental cerebral ischemia in fetal sheep. There is a decrease in oxygen uptake, an increase in glucose uptake, and an increase in lactate output by the brain during ischemia. (From Chao CR, Hohimer AR, Bissonnette JM. Cerebral carbohydrate metabolism during severe ischemia in fetal sheep. J Cerebral Blood Flow Metab 1989; 9:53–57. Reprinted with permission.)

previously implicated in adult and immature individuals. During combined hypoxemia and cerebral ischemia, however, the same group of authors could not detect a net lactate flux. They suggested that this may be due to a concomitant cerebral and systemic increase in lactate concentration.

In a similar model, it was shown that glucose infusion tended to maintain electroencephalographic (EEG) amplitude during cerebral ischemia, thus suggesting it had a protective effective. In further studies, fetal glucose levels were reduced 33 percent by insulin infusion. This did not produce any short-term reduction in cerebral oxygen or glucose consumption (reviewed by Parer[16]).

The presence of adequate brain carbohydrate stores has been demonstrated in the past to be an important determinant of tolerance to asphyxia at birth. Thus the survival time of insulin treated newborn rats was only one tenth that of normoglycemic litter mates when exposed to nitrogen.[28]

## C Asphyxia, Reduced Cerebral Metabolism, and Neuronal Damage

Severe fetal asphyxia can cause cerebral palsy and lesser degrees of neurologic damage, though it is now clear that the proportion of cerebral palsy due to birth asphyxia is relatively small, perhaps less than 10 percent (see Chapter 10). The degree of damage to any individual fetus following severe asphyxia can be quite variable. For example, some fetuses may not survive the episode in utero, others have central damage which results in a surviving newborn with neurologic defects, and still others survive without apparent deficits.

At one end of the scale, we have reasonably good evidence for the limits of fetal tolerance for complete absence of oxygen delivery. Myers[14] showed that following complete cessation of fetal oxygen delivery, hypoxemia and both respiratory and metabolic acidosis occurred rapidly. Intact survival generally did not occur after 10 minutes of oxygen lack. Survivors generally had brain stem lesions, although the patterns of damage were variable. If oxygen delivery was prevented for 25 minutes, fetuses could be resuscitated but apparently the hypoxic damage to numerous organs, including the heart, was so severe that the death occurred within a short time. Myers and his coworkers[14, 25] have also studied prolonged partial asphyxia in sheep and monkeys brought on by a variety of mechanisms. As with brief complete asphyxia they found a variable pattern of response. Survivors generally had neurologic deficits due to cortical lesions, in contrast to those subjected to complete oxygen cessation. Prolonged partial asphyxia in the above studies has been difficult to define, probably because of the several components, such as degree of hypoxemia, duration, and initial condition of the fetus.

There is relatively little information about the relationship between reduced cerebral oxygenation and neuronal cell damage. We have reported cerebral histologic and electrophysiologic changes after asphyxia in chronically instrumented fetal sheep, induced by reducing uterine blood flow to result in an ascending aortic blood oxygen content of less than 1.5 mM.[8] In an initial protocol, asphyxia continued for up to 60 minutes, and in a subsequent study supplementary maternal hypoxia was added if full occlusion of the common uterine artery for 15 minutes did not reduce the EEG voltage to less than 20 percent of baseline.

Uterine artery occlusion resulted in severe hypoxemia, hypercarbia, acidosis, and an initial hypertension and bradycardia. Eight of 14 surviving fetuses showed neuronal damage, with greatest loss in the parasagittal cortex, striatum, and the CA12 region of the hippocampus, after 3 days. Neuronal damage was strongly associated with the minimum blood pressure during the insult but not with the degree of hypoxia (Fig. 5–6). No other factor was independently predictive, but when considered separately the pH at the end of asphyxia and loss of intensity of the EEG were also correlated with outcome. The pH fell to <7.0 in six of eight with damage, while it remained >7.0 in five of six with no damage ($P$ <0.05). We concluded that severe intrauterine asphyxia for periods of 30 to 120 minutes can cause predominantly parasagittal neuronal death, and that this is associated with hypotension, severe metabolic acidosis, and suppression of EEG during the insult.[8] These data are consistent with the suggestion that impairment of cerebral perfusion is a critical event in causing cerebral damage during perinatal asphyxia.[25]

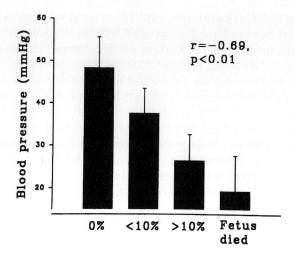

**FIGURE 5–6.** Relationship between minimum blood pressure during severe asphyxia and percentage of dead neurons in the parasaggital cortex (horizontal axis) at 72 hours in fetal sheep. (Modified from Gunn AJ, Parer JT, Mallard EC, et al. Cerebral histologic and electrocorticographic changes after asphyxia in fetal sheep. Pediatr Res 1992; 31:486–491.)

We have measured cerebral oxygen consumption in a further series of fetal sheep using the above protocol.[1] In the animals that subsequently developed seizure activity, the fetal arterial oxygen content fell from $3.0 \pm 0.9$ mM (mean $\pm$ SD) to 0.5 mM. The blood flow to the cerebral cortex during control was $163 \pm 51$ ml $\cdot$ 100 g$^{-1} \cdot$ min$^{-1}$, and increased to 90 percent above control by 30 minutes of asphyxia. It then progressively fell to approach control values by 90 minutes. The arteriovenous oxygen difference narrowed so that cortical oxygen consumption decreased to 36 percent of control. The fetal arterial pH fell from $7.39 \pm 0.03$ to $6.89 \pm 0.01$, the base excess from $4.7 \pm 2.4$ mEq $\cdot$ L$^{-1}$ to $-21.6 \pm 5.7$ mEq $\cdot$ L$^{-1}$, and the carbon dioxide tension rose from $49 \pm 3$ mm Hg to $66 \pm 0$ mm Hg, during the asphyxial insult. Fetuses that survived without seizures generally had lower falls in cortical oxygen consumption. Fetuses that died during or shortly after the insult either had arrhythmias or a rapid progression of asphyxia. These data suggest that depression of oxygen consumption by the fetal cortex to less than 50 percent of control over approximately 90 minutes results in neurologic damage as demonstrated by seizures. Damage to other organs was apparently not sufficient to be lethal within 24 hours.[1]

With respect to another technique for producing fetal asphyxia, Mallard et al.[13] have produced neuronal cell loss in the hippocampus by severe umbilical cord occlusion for 10 minutes in near-term fetal sheep. Although the duration was short, there was severe asphyxia, hypoxemia, bradycardia and electrocorticographic suppression for up to 5 hours. Three of 17 animals did not survive the asphyxia. The metabolism during asphyxia was not quantitated, but it was most likely severely depressed. We have produced seizures after umbilical cord occlusion of lesser severity and for a longer duration.[2]

We do not have data on the exact threshold of reduction in oxygen consumption that causes damage to the fetal brain. It seems likely, however, that a 15 percent reduction would be tolerable. It has been shown that a change in electrocorticographic activity from low-voltage, high-frequency to high-voltage, low-frequency activity is associated with a similar decrease in oxygen uptake.[20] The degree of hypoxemia seen in our moderately asphyxiated fetuses is usually associated with such an EEG change from low to high voltage, and this alone may explain the decrease in cerebral oxygen consumption.

The reduction of cerebral oxygen consumption to approximately 50 percent of control may be associated with further compensatory mechanisms for preventing neuronal damage, but we cannot determine such from our studies. Severe asphyxia in the immediate newborn period has been associated with functional and anatomic central nervous system damage in monkeys,[14] but it is not possible to compare the physiologic conditions of that study with those quoted above.

These studies have some important clinical implications. They show the remarkable conservation strategies available to the fetus despite quite substantial hypoxemia, mainly due to the fetal capacity for augmenting blood flow. This may explain why intact survival is not infrequently seen in the human fetus despite severe documented asphyxia at birth. With profound asphyxia, however, there is decompensation of these mechanisms and such fetuses may subsequently develop hypoxic neuronal damage.

## D Regulation of Cerebral Metabolism During Asphyxia

The fetal brain blood flow is sensitive to changes in oxygen and carbon dioxide, and as noted, metabolic rate is constant over a wide range of oxygen content of perfusing blood, because there is a compensatory balance between the blood flow and arteriovenous oxygen concentration difference (Table 5–3). The CBF is also directly proportional to carbon dioxide tension, but this almost certainly does not result in increased oxygen consumption by the brain. The response may teleologically be thought of as a mechanism for reducing elevated brain carbon dioxide.

The mechanism of the increased CBF in response to either of these mechanisms are unsure. Carbon dioxide has an independent effect, and this

**TABLE 5–3.   Factors Affecting Vascular Resistance and Fetal Cortical Blood Flow During Asphyxia**

Oxygen content
Carbon dioxide tension
Adenosine
Arginine vasopressin
Prostaglandins
Nitric oxide
Loss of autoregulation

may alter the brain's ability to tolerate hypoxia, because as carbon dioxide falls, CBF also falls, and in order to maintain oxygen consumption, oxygen extraction must increase. During hypoxia this may be limited, so oxygen consumption may fall.[9] This is of less importance in the fetus because during asphyxia in utero carbon dioxide almost invariably rises, unless there is extreme maternal hyperventilation.

There are several possible mechanisms for the variations in CBF during hypoxia, and one possibility (extrapolating from adult studies) is a direct action of oxygen tension on smooth muscle. Oxygenases have been suggested as oxygen sensors in mediating the responses. Release of the vasodilator adenosine may be one such mechanism. It has been shown that brain vascular resistance increases and CBF decreases during hypoxia in fetal sheep in response to arginine vasopressin, prostaglandin, and nitric oxide[27] blockade, thus demonstrating a role for these substances. There may also be other as yet unidentified substances and mechanisms (reviewed in Parer[16]).

**TABLE 5–4.   Cerebral Metabolism in Fetal Sheep: Miscellaneous Factors**

Anesthesia and drugs
    Halothane: no change during asphyxia
    Isofluorane: no change during asphyxia
    Pentobarbital: 27% reduction
    Ethanol: 23% reduction in near term fetuses
            no change in immature fetuses (0.6 gestation)
Status epilepticus
    Initial four- to eight-fold increase in newborn primates
Increased intracranial pressure (infusion into ventricle)
    No change in oxygen uptake (due to increased blood pressure and CBF)

See Parer[16] for sources of data.

# E   Miscellaneous Factors Affecting Cerebral Metabolism[16] (Table 5–4)

## ANESTHESIA AND DRUGS

Pentobarbital resulted in a 27 percent decrease in cerebral oxygen consumption at constant perfusion pressure in normoxemic fetal sheep. During hypoxia, with barbiturate treatment, there were still increases in CBF, but in proportion to the reduced metabolism. Similar studies with both halothane and isofluorane-oxygen in fetal sheep demonstrated retention of the ability of the fetal cerebral circulations to vasodilate during asphyxia.

Ethanol infusion resulted in a 23 percent reduction of cerebral oxygen consumption in near-term fetal sheep. The dosage was selected to mimic episodic binge-type drinking in humans. The authors concluded that the reduced cerebral metabolism represented a direct depressant effect on tissue (e.g., protein or DNA) synthesis and an indirect effect on fetal states. This may explain growth abnormalities in infants exposed to large doses of alcohol in utero.

In contrast to this, alcohol administration to more immature sheep fetuses had little influence on cerebral oxidative or carbohydrate metabolic rates. The difference between the responses of the mature and immature fetuses remains unexplained.

## STATUS EPILEPTICUS

Oxygen consumption by the brain is known to increase in the adult during generalized seizures. Local glucose cerebral metabolism has been studied in newborn primates, and increased up to four- to eightfold in the cortex. The latter authors noted that after 45 minutes of seizures the glucose uptake fell twofold, probably because energy demand exceeded glucose supply.

## INCREASED INTRACRANIAL PRESSURE

Increased intracranial pressure caused by infusion of fluid into the lateral ventricle caused an increase in arterial blood pressure, and maintenance of perfusion pressure, which resulted in maintenance of CBF. There was a concomitant decrease in visceral blood flow. There was thus maintenance of cerebral oxygen consumption during this simulated "head compression," possibly mediated by increases in epinephrine, norepinephrine, and arginine vasopressin.

## REFERENCES

**1.** Ball RH, Espinoza MI, Parer JT, et al. Cerebral blood flow and metabolism in asphyxiated fetuses resulting in seizures. J Matern Fetal Med 1994; 3:157–162.

2. Ball RH, Parer JT, Caldwell LE, Johnson J. Regional blood flow and metabolism in ovine fetuses during severe cord occlusion. Am J Obstet Gynecol 1994; 171:1549–1555.

3. Chao CR, Hohimer AR, Bissonnette JM. Cerebral carbohydrate metabolism during severe ischemia in fetal sheep. J Cerebral Blood Flow Metab 1989; 9:53–57.

4. Cohn HE, Sacks EJ, Heymann MA, Rudolph AM. Cardiovascular responses to hypoxemia and acidemia in fetal lambs. Am J Obstet Gynecol 1974; 120:817–824.

5. Field DR, Parer JT, Auslender RA, et al. Cerebral oxygen consumption during asphyxia in fetal sheep. J Dev Physiol 1990; 14:131–137.

6. Gleason CA, Hamm C, Jones MD Jr. Cerebral blood flow, oxygenation, and carbohydrate metabolism in immature fetal sheep in utero. Am J Physiol 1989; 256(6):R1264–R1268.

7. Gleason CA, Hamm C, Jones MD Jr. Effect of acute hypoxemia on brain blood flow and oxygen metabolism in immature fetal sheep. Am J Physiol 1990; 258 (Heart Circ Physiol 27):H1064–H1069.

8. Gunn AJ, Parer JT, Mallard EC, et al. Cerebral histologic and electrocorticographic changes after asphyxia in fetal sheep. Pediatr Res 1992; 31:486–491.

9. Jones MD Jr, Rosenberg AA, Simmons MA, et al. Oxygen delivery to the brain before and after birth. Science 1982; 216:324–325.

10. Jones MD Jr, Sheldon RE, Peeters LL, et al. Regulation of cerebral blood flow in the ovine fetus. Am J Physiol 1978; 235:H162–H166.

11. Jones MD Jr, Sheldon RE, Peeters LL, et al. Fetal cerebral oxygen consumption at different levels of oxygenation. J Appl Physiol: Respir Environ Exercise Physiol 1977; 43(6):1080–1084.

12. Jones MD Jr, Traystman RJ. Cerebral oxygenation of the fetus, newborn, and adult. Semin Perinatol 1984; 8:205–216.

13. Mallard EC, Gunn AJ, Williams CE, et al. Transient umbilical cord occlusion causes hippocampal damage in the fetal sheep. Am J Obstet Gynecol 1992; 167:1423–1430.

14. Myers RE. Two patterns of perinatal brain damage and their conditions of occurrence. Am J Obstet Gynecol 1972; 112:246–276.

15. Papile L-A, Rudolph AM, Heyman MA. Autoregulation of cerebral blood flow in preterm fetal lamb. Pediatr Res 1985; 19:159–161.

16. Parer JT. Fetal cerebral metabolism: The influence of asphyxia and other factors. J Perinatol 1994; 14:376–385.

17. Peeters LLH, Sheldon RE, Jones MD, et al. Blood flow to fetal organs as a function of arterial oxygen content. Am J Obstet Gynecol 1979; 135:637–646.

18. Purves MJ, James IM. Observations on the control of cerebral blood flow in the sheep fetus and newborn lamb. Circ Res 1969; 25:651–667.

19. Richardson BS. The effect of behavioral state on fetal metabolism and blood flow circulation. Semin Perinatol 1992; 16:227–233.

20. Richardson BS, Patrick JE, Abduljabbar H. Cerebral oxidative metabolism in the fetal lamb: Relationship to electrocortical state. Am J Obstet Gynecol 1985; 153:426–431.

21. Richardson BS, Rurak D, Patrick JE, et al. Cerebral oxidative metabolism during sustained hypoxaemia in fetal sheep. J Dev Physiol 1989; 11:37–43.

22. Rosenberg AA, Jones MD Jr, Traystman RJ, et al. Response of cerebral blood flow to changes in $P_{CO_2}$ in fetal, newborn, and adult sheep. Am J Physiol 1982; 242:H862–H866.

**23.** Sokoloff L. Relationships among local functional activity, energy metabolism, and blood flow in the central nervous system. Fed Proc 1981; 40:2311–2316.

**24.** Szymonowicz W, Walker AM, Cussen L, et al. Developmental changes in regional cerebral blood flow in fetal and newborn lambs. Am J Physiol 1988; 254:H52–H58.

**25.** Ting P, Yamaguchi S, Bacher JD, et al. Hypoxic-ischemic cerebral necrosis in midgestational sheep fetuses: Physiopathologic correlations. Exp Neurol 1983; 80:227–245.

**26.** Tweed WA, Cote J, Pash M, Lou H. Arterial oxygenation determines autoregulation of cerebral blood flow in the fetal lamb. Pediatr Res 1983; 17:246–249.

**27.** Van Bel F, Sola A, Roman C, Rudolph AM. Role of nitric oxide in the regulation of the cerebral circulation in the lamb fetus during normoxemia and hypoxemia. Biol Neonate 1995; 68:200–210.

**28.** Vannucci RC, Vannucci SJ. Cerebral carbohydrate metabolism during hypoglycemia and anoxia in newborn rats. Ann Neurol 1978; 4:73–79.

# ■ *Chapter Six*

# Acid-Base Physiology

In this chapter, acid-base balance[3] and normal maternal and fetal blood values are described. Placental exchange of carbon dioxide has been covered in Chapter 3, and the technique of fetal blood sampling and its use with other ancillary techniques will be described in Chapter 8.

## I ACIDS PRODUCED BY THE BODY

The body has mechanisms that attempt to maintain the hydrogen ion concentration (symbolized as $[H^+]$) within narrow limits, so that the cellular biochemical reactions may occur optimally.

The body produces two groups of acids: carbonic and noncarbonic.

## A Carbonic Acid

Carbonic acid is formed by hydration of carbon dioxide, which results from oxidative metabolism. Carbon dioxide is primarily regulated in the adult by alveolar ventilation, which normally is set to maintain a level of carbon dioxide pressure of 40 mmHg in the alveoli (and arterial blood). As will be seen later in this discussion, pregnant women have a level set below this, 34 mmHg. Normally, the fetus rapidly disposes of carbon dioxide across the placenta by diffusion into the maternal blood. This process requires adequate blood flow on each side of the placenta (i.e., intervillous flow on the maternal side and umbilical flow on the fetal side).

## B  Noncarbonic Acid

There are several noncarbonic (metabolic or fixed) acids: lactic, β-hydroxybutyric, and other organic acids. Lactic acid can be utilized in aerobic metabolism (the Krebs, or citric acid cycle), and it is also a major end product of anaerobic glycolysis, which is a temporary mechanism by which the body produces high-energy phosphate molecules such as adenosine triphosphate (ATP), even in the absence of oxygen. It is far less efficient than the aerobic cycle, since only two ATP molecules are formed per molecule of glucose, compared with 38 ATP molecules per molecule of glucose in the aerobic cycle. Beta-hydroxybutyric acid is produced during fat breakdown (e.g., in starvation or in diabetic ketoacidosis).

In the adult, these fixed acids are regulated by renal excretion, and their removal is slower than that of carbon dioxide (i.e., under appropriate conditions disposal takes hours rather than seconds). The fetus is able to dispose of the fixed acids across the placenta, and diffusion of these acids is similarly far slower than that of carbon dioxide. An alternative means of disposal of lactate is by metabolism if oxygenation becomes adequate. This process also is relatively slow compared with carbon dioxide diffusion.

  LIMITS OF ACIDITY COMPATIBLE WITH SURVIVAL

The acidity of body fluids can be expressed either as the concentration of the hydrogen ion or, in a more manageable form, as pH. The term *pH* comes from the French *puissance hydrogène;* it is the negative logarithm to the base 10 of [H⁺]. Thus, [H⁺] of $10^{-7}$ mol $\cdot$ L⁻¹ is equivalent to a pH of 7. The normal [H⁺] in adult blood plasma is $40 \times 10^{-9}$ mol $\cdot$ L⁻¹, which corresponds to a pH of 7.4.

The generally accepted limits of acidity compatible with survival are $160 \times 10^{-9}$ to $20 \times 10^{-9}$ mol $\cdot$ L⁻¹, or pH of 6.8 to 7.7.

## A  The Henderson–Hasselbalch Equation

The pH of blood at any moment will depend on the proportion of carbonic and fixed acids present. Chemically, it has been shown that

$$[H^+] = K \frac{[acid]}{[base]}$$

where K is a constant for a particular acid and the concentrations of acid and base are measured. This relationship is changed to negative logarithm notation for convenience:

$$-\log [H^+] = -\log K + \log \frac{[\text{base}]}{[\text{acid}]}$$

The Henderson–Hasselbalch equation is thus:

$$pH = pK + \log \frac{[\text{base}]}{[\text{acid}]}$$

For the acid-base pair, carbonic acid and bicarbonate ($H_2CO_3 \rightarrow H^+ + HCO_3^-$) the pK is 6.1. The bicarbonate concentration [$HCO_3^-$] in blood is normally 24 mM $\cdot$ L$^{-1}$, and the normal value of [$H_2CO_3$] is 1.2 mM $\cdot$ L$^{-1}$. The latter value can be calculated from the carbon dioxide pressure (normally 40 mmHg) multiplied by the solubility constant for carbon dioxide, 0.03.

Hence, the normal pH can be calculated as

$$pH = pK + \frac{[HCO_3^-]}{[H_2CO_3]}$$
$$= 6.1 + \log \tfrac{24}{1.2}$$
$$= 6.1 + \log 20$$
$$= 6.1 + 1.3$$
$$= 7.4$$

It should be noted that a change in either the carbon dioxide pressure or the bicarbonate concentration will alter the pH. Increasing the carbon dioxide pressure (e.g., by hypoventilation) will cause the pH to fall (respiratory acidosis). Decreasing the bicarbonate concentration (e.g., by accumulation of lactic acid) will cause the pH to fall (metabolic acidosis).

If any two of the three factors in the Henderson–Hasselbalch equation are known, the third can be calculated. In clinical practice, pH and carbon dioxide pressure are measured, and the bicarbonate is calculated from the Henderson–Hasselbalch equation or, more commonly, from the nomogram constructed from it (Fig. 6–1). Blood gas machines in common use today have inbuilt microprocessors whereby the bicarbonate and base excess are automatically calculated and displayed.

## B  Base Excess

The bicarbonate concentration can change in two ways: It may react with fixed acids, and it will vary with changes in carbon dioxide content because of buffering of carbonic acid by hemoglobin. Because of this variation, the bicarbonate concentration is only of value for determining the degree of derangement of metabolic activity when carbon dioxide pressure is normal (i.e., 40 mmHg). Hence, the concept of base excess was introduced as a measure of magnitude of the metabolic acid-base change (i.e., bicarbonate)

# SIGGAARD-ANDERSEN ALIGNMENT NOMOGRAM

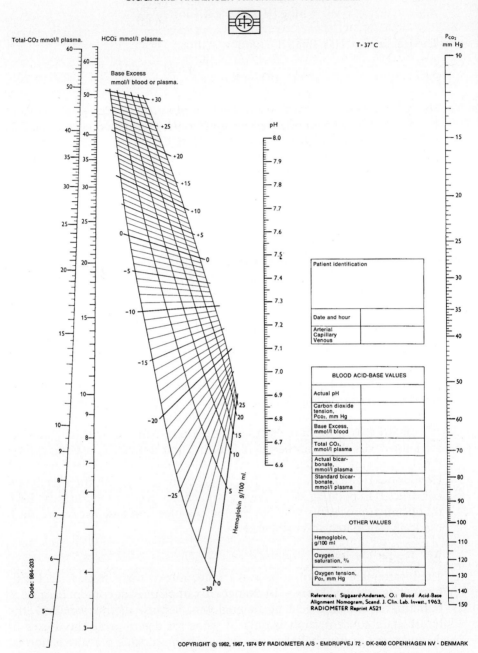

**FIGURE 6–1.**    A nomogram relating blood carbon dioxide tension and pH to plasma bicarbonate and base excess. (From Siggaard-Andersen O. Blood acid-base alignment nomogram. Scand J Clin Lab Invest 1963. Used by permission.)

from normal, even in the presence of a concomitant respiratory (i.e., carbon dioxide pressure) change.

Base excess is calculated from known measured values of pH and carbon dioxide tension by means of a nomogram (Fig. 6–1) or a special slide rule. A small correction may be made for variations in hemoglobin concentration. However, the value is conventionally read at a hemoglobin of $5 \; g \cdot dl^{-1}$, because this is a better approximation after whole-body equilibration. Base deficit is the same as base excess, except that the sign is changed.

## III  NORMAL VALUES

Normal adult values of acid-base factors in arterial blood are presented in Table 6–1.

The pregnant woman's pH is normal, but she hyperventilates to such a degree that her alveolar (and arterial blood) carbon dioxide pressure is reduced to approximately 34 mmHg. It is thought that progesterone is responsible for this hyperventilation, because administration of this hormone to male subjects can induce hyperventilation. Hyperventilation also correlates with progesterone levels during the menstrual cycle. The pH is normal because of the excretion of bicarbonate, which is regulated by the kidneys. The pregnant woman is thus in a state of compensated respiratory alkalosis.

Approximations of normal values of acid-base state and blood gases in relatively undisturbed human blood were obtained from fetal capillary blood samples before the onset of labor. From these values, and those obtained from chronically catheterized fetal animals (mainly sheep), it was suspected that the acid-base state was very close to that of the mother (Table 6–2). The major difference is that the carbon dioxide tension is somewhat higher in order to provide a gradient for carbon dioxide diffusion across the placenta. Similar measurements during labor showed that the fetus developed a mild respiratory and metabolic acidosis by the second stage of labour.

TABLE 6–1.  **Normal Adult Arterial Blood Acid-Base Values**

|  | *Nonpregnant* | *Pregnant* |
|---|---|---|
| pH | 7.40 | 7.40 |
| Carbon dioxide pressure (mmHg) | 40 | 34 |
| Bicarbonate (mEq $\cdot$ $L^{-1}$) | 24 | 21 |
| Base excess (mEq $\cdot$ $L^{-1}$) | 0 | −4 |

**TABLE 6–2.   Average Fetal Scalp Blood Acid-Base Values**

|  | Before Labor | Second Stage of Labor |
|---|---|---|
| pH | 7.37 | 7.30 |
| Carbon dioxide pressure (mmHg) | 38 | 43 |
| Bicarbonate (mEq $\cdot$ L$^{-1}$) | 21 | 21 |
| Base excess (mEq $\cdot$ L$^{-1}$) | −3 | −5 |

Modified from Rooth G, Jacobson L, Heinrich J, Seidenschnur G. The acid-base status of the fetus during normal labor. In Longo LD, Bartels H, eds. Respiratory Gas Exchange and Blood Flow in the Placenta. U.S. Department of Health, Education and Welfare Publications, Bethesda, MD, 1972, pp. 477–486.

Umbilical arterial and venous blood gas samples in relatively undisturbed third-trimester human fetuses were not available until the advent of fetoscopy and cordocentesis (Table 6–3). The mean values are close to those of the adult, but the range of "normal" appears to be greater.[4]

There is a great deal more known about acid-base state and blood gases in umbilical cord vessels at the time of delivery. As noted above, a mild mixed respiratory and metabolic acidosis develops during labor. It is so common and so minor, however, that it is considered to be a normal physiologic event of no harmful significance to the fetus. Mean values for umbilical artery and vein blood gases at birth have been obtained on a number of large series of hundreds of "normal" births, and the range is ever greater than that in utero before labor.[1, 2, 5] In Table 6–4, the results of one analysis of over 15,000 newborns is shown.[1] All had Apgar scores ≥7 at 5 minutes. The mean pH was

**TABLE 6–3.   Acid-Base and Blood Gas Values in Umbilical Cord Vessels in the In Utero Human Fetus at Approximately 35 Weeks' Gestation**

|  | Umbilical Artery | Umbilical Vein |
|---|---|---|
| pH | 7.33 ± 0.07[a] | 7.38 ± 0.06 |
| Carbon dioxide pressure (mmHg) | 45 ± 10 | 38 ± 8 |
| Bicarbonate (mEq $\cdot$ L$^{-1}$) | 23 ± 5 | 23 ± 5 |
| Base excess (mEq $\cdot$ L$^{-1}$) | −3 ± 3 | +0.5 ± 4 |
| Oxygen content (mM $\cdot$ L$^{-1}$) | — | 6.7 ± 0.6 |
| Oxygen pressure (mmHg) | 35 ± 15 | 41 ± 20 |
| Hemoglobin (g $\cdot$ dl$^{-1}$) | 13 | 13 |

[a]Mean ± 2 SD.

n = ≥50.

Modified from Nicolaides KH, Kypros HN, Rodeck CH, Campbell S. Effect of gestational age on fetal and intervillous blood gas and acid-base values in human pregnancy. Fetal Therapy 1986; 1:168–175.

**TABLE 6–4.** Mean and Median Values of Acid-Base and Blood Gas Values in Umbilical Arterial (UA) and Venous (UV) Cord Blood in Fetuses with Apgar Score ≥7 at 5 Minutes

|  | Mean | Std Dev | 2.5 %tile | 5th %tile | Median | 95th %tile | 97.5 %tile |
|---|---|---|---|---|---|---|---|
| UA pH | 7.26 | 0.07 | 7.10 | 7.13 | 7.27 | 7.36 | 7.38 |
| UA $pCO_2$ (mmHg) | 53 | 10 | 35 | 37 | 52 | 69 | 74 |
| UA $pO_2$ (mmHg) | 17 | 6 | 6 | 8 | 17 | 27 | 30 |
| UA base excess (mEq • $L^{-1}$) | −4 | 3 | −11 | −10 | −4 | 1 | 1 |
| UV pH | 7.34 | 0.06 | 7.20 | 7.23 | 7.35 | 7.44 | 7.46 |
| UV $pCO_2$ (mmHg) | 41 | 7 | 28 | 30 | 41 | 53 | 57 |
| UV $pO_2$ (mmHg) | 29 | 7 | 16 | 18 | 29 | 40 | 43 |
| UV base excess (mEq • $L^{-1}$) | −3 | 3 | −8 | −8 | −3 | 1 | 2 |

$pCO_2$, carbon dioxide pressure; $pO_2$, oxygen pressure.

n = 15,073.

From Helwig JT, Parer JT, Kilpatrick SJ, Laros RK Jr. Umbilical cord blood acid base state: What is normal? Am J Obstet Gynecol. 174:1807–1814. 1996. Used by permission.

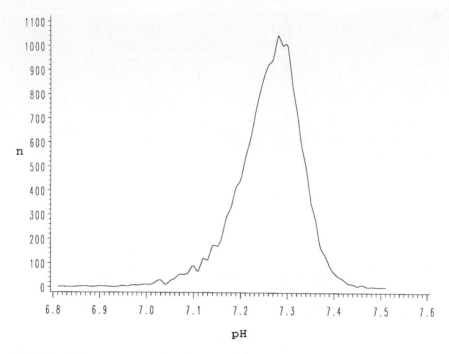

**FIGURE 6–2.**   Frequency distribution of umbilical arterial pH in 15,073 preterm and term babies born vaginally or by cesarean section with Apgar scores ≥7 at 5 minutes. The skewness is toward acidosis. The shape of the curve and skewness remains the same if the values are expressed as hydrogen ion concentration. (From Helwig JT, Parer JT, Kilpatrick SJ, Laros RK Jr. Umbilical cord blood acid base state: What is normal? Am J Obstet Gynecol, 174:1807–1814, 1996. Used with permission.)

7.26, and the lower limits of normal for umbilical artery pH and base excess expressed as the 2.5th percentile in such normal babies are 7.10 and $-11 \ mEq \cdot 1^{-1}$, respectively. A frequency distribution of the pH values is shown in Figure 6–2. A further discussion of these values, and the concept of asphyxia sufficient to cause tissue damage, will be found in Chapter 10.

## REFERENCES

**1.** Helwig JT, Parer JT, Kilpatrick SJ, Laros RK Jr. Umbilical cord blood acid base state: What is normal? Am J Obstet Gynecol 1996; 1704:1807–1814.

**2.** Riley RJ, Johnson JWC. Collecting and analyzing cord blood gases. Clin Obstet Gynecol 1993; 36:13–23.

**3.** Shapiro BA, Peruzzi WT, Templin R. Clinical Application of Blood Gases, 5th ed. Mosby–Year Book, St. Louis, 1994.

**4.** Soothill PW, Nicolaides HN, Rodeck CH, Campbell S. Effect of gestational age on fetal and intervillous blood gas and acid-base values in human pregnancy. Fetal Therapy 1986; 1:168–175.

**5.** Sykes GS, Johnson P, Ashworth F, et al. Do Apgar scores indicate asphyxia? Lancet 1982; 1:494–496.

# Part Three

# INSTRUMENTATION
# AND TECHNIQUES

# ■ *Chapter Seven*

# The Fetal Heart Rate Monitor

The fetal heart rate (FHR) monitor is a device with two components: one to recognize and process heart rate and the other to identify uterine contractions[3] (Fig. 7–1). Full technical descriptions of the devices can be found in the service manuals and operating guides provided by the manufacturers.

For recognition of the FHR, the device can use the R-wave of the fetal electrocardiogram (ECG) complex, a signal generated by the movement of a cardiovascular structure, using ultrasound and the Doppler principle, or cardiac sounds by means of a microphone pickup. Uterine contractions are detected either by a catheter inserted transcervically into the amniotic cavity and attached to a strain-gauge transducer, or by an external device, termed a *tokodynamometer,* which is placed on the maternal abdomen and which recognizes the tightening of the maternal abdomen during a contraction.

Monitoring with devices that are attached directly to the fetus or placed within the uterine cavity is called *direct, internal,* or *invasive* monitoring. The fetal electrode (generally a stainless-steel spiral) and the intraamniotic catheter are examples of direct monitoring equipment. Devices that do not require direct connection with the fetus are called *noninvasive* or *external.* They consist of the Doppler ultrasound device, the phonocardiogram or the external abdominal ECG for detecting heart rate, and the tokodynamometer for sensing uterine contractions. In current clinical practice, in external monitoring the Doppler device is almost always used for detecting the FHR. The most accurate apparatus for detecting heart rate is that which gives the most discrete signal and has the least external interference. Monitoring the R-wave of the fetal ECG complex is the most accurate method in the intrapartum period, although as noted below, modern Doppler devices can usually give a perfectly adequate signal.

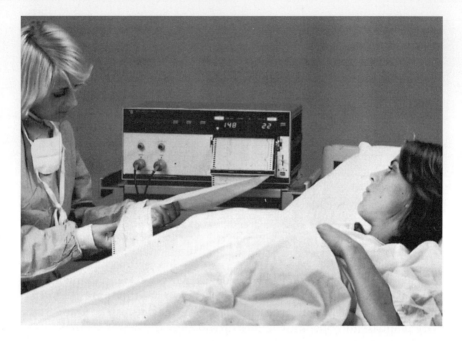

**FIGURE 7–1.** An example of a commercially available FHR monitor, with recording being made during labor. (Courtesy of Hewlett Packard Company, Palo Alto, California.)

A critical component of the fetal monitor is the cardiotachometer. An understanding of its mode of action is essential for appreciating FHR variability. Within the monitor is a device for recognizing the cardiac event. Another component measures the time interval between the events, and a third device rapidly divides the time interval in seconds into 60 to give a rate for each interval between beats. These individual rates then are traced on a strip chart recorder, which moves at a specific speed. Examples of several heart beats and the resulting recordings are shown in Figure 7–2. When the paper moves slowly, instead of having a plateau-like pattern as shown in the illustration at fast paper speed, the recordings appear as a jittery line; this pattern is described as *variability*. If each interval between heart beats were identical, then the line would be flat. This phenomenon is termed *absent variability*, or a flat or silent baseline. The ability of the various devices to depict variability accurately is dependent on the discreteness of the signal that is portraying cardiac events and the accuracy with which the event can be detected.

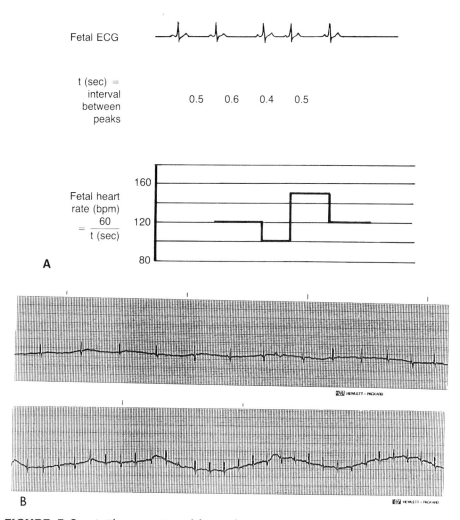

**FIGURE 7–2.** A. The operation of the cardiotachometer. The peaks of the R-waves are detected, and the time interval between them is measured. This measurement is electronically divided into 60, and the resulting rate is traced on a strip chart recorder. This example shows the usual situation, in which there are slight differences between adjacent heart beats, giving rise to heart rate variability. B. Electrocardiogram tracings from a fetus recorded a few minutes apart, showing a deceleration of approximately 60 beats/min above and a normal rate of approximately 150 beats/min below.

# I  FETAL HEART RATE

## A  Fetal Electrode

Currently, the internal means of detecting FHR consists almost exclusively of a small stainless-steel spiral electrode that is attached to the fetal scalp (Fig. 7–3). The second contact is bathed by vaginal fluids. The wires traverse the vaginal canal and are connected to the machine, in which the data are processed and the FHR is displayed. This mode gives the most valid FHR tracing because of the discreteness of the signal; therefore, it best depicts beat-to-beat variability.

Placement of the spiral electrode on the fetus is facilitated by a rigid plastic tube enclosing another tube, the electrode holder. This apparatus is

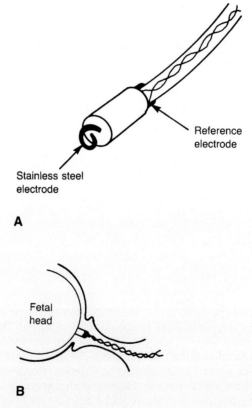

Reference electrode

Stainless steel electrode

A

Fetal head

B

**FIGURE 7–3.**   A. The spiral electrode, for directly recording the fetal ECG. B. A sagittal section showing attachment of the spiral to the fetal scalp and the wires traversing the cervix and vagina.

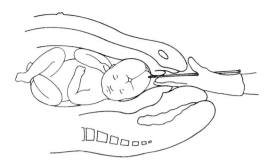

**FIGURE 7–4.**  Technique for placement of the spiral electrode.

placed against the fetal scalp over a bony area (not the suture line or fontanelle), and a 360 degree motion of the electrode holder results in the attachment of the steel spiral to the scalp (Fig. 7–4). The spiral is approximately 2 mm deep, and the skull is at least 3 mm below the surface of the scalp, so the electrode is in soft tissue only. It also may be placed over the gluteal area in a breech presentation. It should never be placed on the face (for cosmetic reasons) or on an undiagnosed presentation. The electrode almost always can be inserted after cervical dilatation of about 2 cm. The membranes should be ruptured or will be ruptured by the act of placing the electrode.

This mode frequently is preferred by patients, because it allows a certain amount of mobility and position choice and does not require abdominal belts.

## B  The Doppler Ultrasound Transducer

This apparatus consists of a device that is affixed to the maternal abdominal wall and transmits a high-frequency ultrasoundsound of approximately 2.5 MHz (Fig. 7–5). The signal is reflected from a moving structure (e.g., the ventricle wall) and the reflected beam is changed in frequency, depending on whether the wall moved away from or toward the source. It is similar to the rise and fall in pitch of a locomotive whistle as a train comes toward, and then passes, a listener. This change in frequency with each systole is recognized as a cardiac event and is processed by the machine.

Although this device is simple to apply and can be used before rupture of the membranes, it sometimes is unreliable during labor because of maternal and fetal movement. A greater disadvantage is that it may not always give a valid indication of beat-to-beat variability, because the Doppler signal is broad and slurred, and the machine is not always able to select accurately and consistently a point on this slurred curve to represent the exact time of a

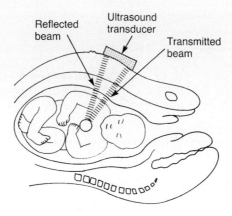

**FIGURE 7–5.**   The Doppler ultrasound device for detecting cardiac activity. The frequency of the reflected beam is changed when it is reflected from a moving structure.

cardiac event (Fig. 7–6). Hence, an artificial short-term variability can be portrayed by the apparatus. Long-term variability, however, may be displayed reasonably accurately (see Chapter 9).

   Improvements in construction and logic have made the later-generation Doppler devices more accurate and easier to use.[1, 2] In particular, the technique of autocorrelation can be used to more accurately define the timing of the cardiac contraction by taking a number of points on the "curve" depicting the Doppler frequency shift. Earlier systems selected a threshold or peak of the curve, thereby making small errors in the timing of the contraction, which resulted in the artifactual "variability" noted

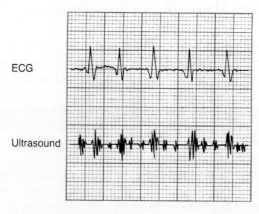

**FIGURE 7–6.**   Contrast between the sharp, discrete signal of the R-wave of the fetal ECG and the slurred ultrasound signal from the moving cardiac structures.

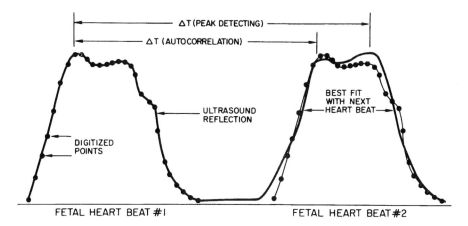

**FIGURE 7–7.** Waveforms of two ultrasound cardiac signals compare integration (peak-to-peak) of the first-generation electronic fetal monitor with autocorrelation of the second-generation electronic fetal monitor. (From Hewlett Packard Company, Palo Alto, California. Used by permission.)

above. In the autocorrelation technique successive heart signals are com-pared and tested for their similarity. Thus, not one point on time within a heart action (the "peak," or "threshold"), but the total waveform complex is compared to the following one (Fig. 7–7).

There is still, however, a problem remaining with the external Doppler detection of the cardiac interval, and that is movement artefact, which will also tend to artifactually increase apparent beat-to-beat variability. To over-come this, an average buffer with several weighted heart beats is built up and the most probable heart rate is generated. This gives the advantage of more easily picking up heart activity, but limits (decreases) beat-to-beat accuracy, particularly during rapid changes of the heart rate.[4]

This smoothing is not so pronounced as that seen with some earlier first-generation monitors, where in order to achieve an acceptably artifact-free tracing, the machines took a running average of two or three beats when in the Doppler mode. In addition to smoothing, this method may have resulted in artificially counting a second heart motion at slow heart rates, thereby doubling the rate. Furthermore, in order to limit detection of a second beat too soon, these machines did not respond to a motion for a fixed period of time, which may have resulted in ignoring every other beat, so that a fast heart rate would be halved.

The ultrasound transducer is best applied to the maternal abdomen over the fetal heart, which is generally subumbilical in the vertex presentation. The best signal generally will be the more discrete movements of the ventricular walls or the valve leaflet motions. Many patients think they are hearing the baby's heart sounds; in fact, they are listening to a frequency shift in the reflected ultrasound, which is translated into sound for convenience.

In searching for the best signal, one should move the transducer slowly rather than with jerking movements, because the ultrasound beam, several centimeters below the transducer, must be reflected from the moving structure.

Some type of coupler gel is applied between transducer and skin for an optimal signal, and the device is held in place by an elastic belt or net placed around the maternal abdomen. As labor progresses or as the mother moves, adjustment of the transducer is needed to retain the optimal signal.

## C The External Abdominal ECG

This device consists of three electrodes placed on the maternal abdomen and records both maternal and fetal ECG complexes. The maternal signal is blanked out, and the remaining fetal signals are used to process heart rate data. An advantage of this apparatus is that it can reflect beat-to-beat variability more accurately than can the other external equipment. Sometimes, however, the maternal and fetal signals coincide, and both will be blanked out. The machine logic will then insert an artificial signal, so this is a source of inaccuracy.

The device is technically more difficult to use than Doppler devices, so experience is required. The external abdominal ECG mode can be used successfully with approximately 80 percent of patients at term but is subject to much artifact during labor because of maternal muscle movement. In addition, the voltage characteristics of the fetal ECG in the period 28 to 34 gestational weeks are such that accurate signals frequently cannot be obtained. Its most important application was in accurately determining FHR variability in antepartum FHR testing, but with the availability of autocorrelation Doppler devices it finds little use today.

## D Phonocardiogram

This device detects fetal heart sounds but rarely is used during labor because of noise artifact. It does give accurate signals in the antepartum period, however. Because of the difficulty in building adequate logic into the phonotransducer, the Doppler method has supplanted it.

## E Sources of Artefact and Error

Fetal heart rate records can be misinterpreted for a number of reasons: (1) electrical or signal defects, (2) limitations of the machinery, or (3) errors of interpretation of the records. The possible sources of error are listed in Table 7–1, together with means of recognizing or solving the problems, and are illustrated by Figures 7–8 to 7–16.

*Text continued on page 113*

**TABLE 7–1.    Sources of Artifact or Error in Fetal Heart Rate Monitoring**

| Source of Error | Solution |
|---|---|
| **Electrical or signal error** | |
| Faulty electrode material, legplate, or monitor | Replace defective parts |
| Improper transducer placement (Fig. 7–8) | Use fetal ECG |
| Intrinsic ECG voltage may be too low | Use Doppler method |
| 60-cycle interference | Grounding |
| Interference by maternal signal | Recognize, and use alternative |
| Maternal ECG | method |
| Maternal muscle movement | |
| Uterine contractions (Fig. 7–9) | |
| Bedpans, and so forth | |
| **Limitations of machinery** | |
| The logic of certain machines may omit FHR that is more than 30 beats/min different from the preceding beat, so may omit arrhythmias | Auscultation can usually detect arrhythmias |
| Averaging—may smooth variability | Recognize that some ultrasound monitors take an average of two or three beats; use fetal ECG if improved trace needed |
| Halving, doubling—very slow rates may be doubled (Figs. 7–10, 7–11), and very high rates (>240 beats/min) may be halved (Fig. 7–12) | Auscultation, to determine correct rate |
| "Short-term variability" in Doppler method caused by indistinct FHR signal (Fig. 7–13) | Realize that one cannot always consistently determine short-term variability with Doppler method |
| **Interpretative errors** | |
| Maternal signal in case of dead fetus (Fig. 7–14) | Compare with maternal rate |
| Maternal signal—electrode on cervix | Compare with maternal rate |
| Scaling errors—two speeds are possible on some machines (1 and 3 cm/min) Fig. 7–15 | Recognize that "patterns" change with rate and use one standard rate, preferably 3 cm/min |
| In Europe, a common "fast" paper speed is 2 cm/min | |
| Nonrecognition of artifact (e.g., "good" variability may be noisy signal, especially with Doppler method) (Fig. 7–13) | Recognize and use alternative method (e.g., fetal ECG) |
| Arrhythmias (tend to be regular) may be confused with artifact (tends to be irregular) (Figs. 7–8, 7–16) | Record fetal ECG from back of machine |

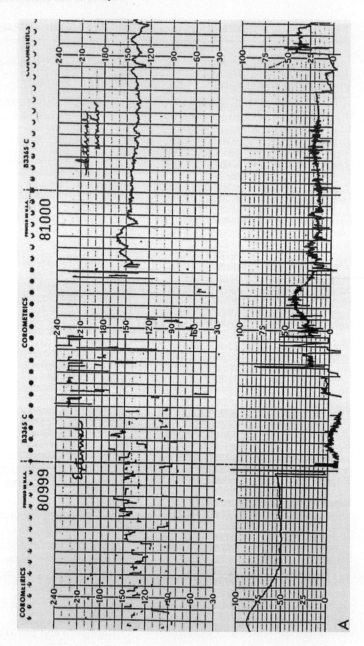

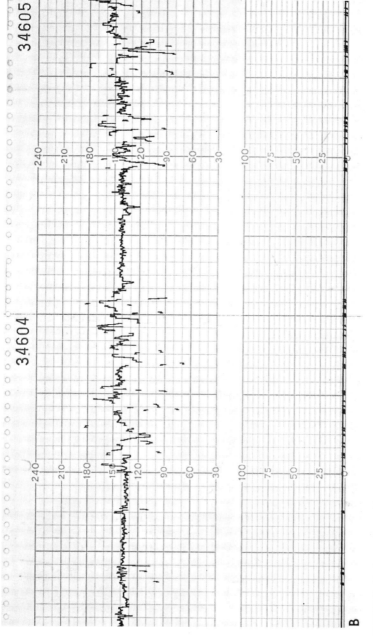

**FIGURE 7–8.** A. Fetal heart rate tracing containing primarily artifacts during the first half of the tracing, using Doppler mode. Note the wide, irregular sweeps of the pen. The internal mode (second half) gives an accurate record. The uterine activity channel is improperly adjusted. B. Episodes of artifact are seen near the center and end of this Doppler recording.

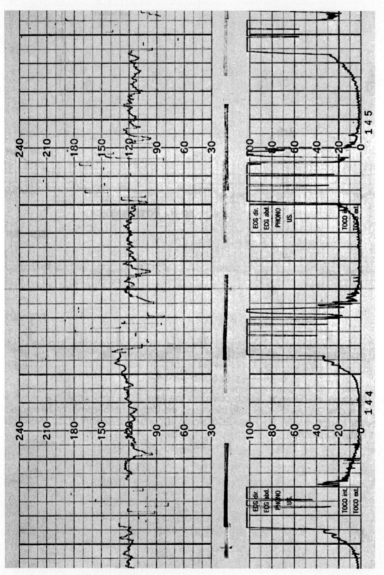

**FIGURE 7–9.** Loss of FHR signal during contractions and maternal "pushing." This phenomenon could be a result of movement of the fetus away from the ultrasound beam (Doppler mode), electrical activity from muscle movement, or poor contact of the reference electrode (see Figure 7–3) during crowning of the head (internal electrode).

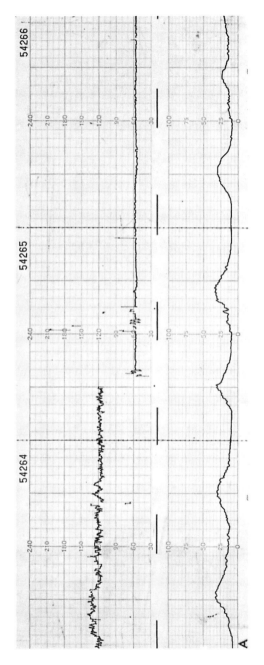

**FIGURE 7–10.**    Possible doubling of a slow rate by the ultrasound device is shown in first half of tracing. This fetus had complete heart block with a ventricular rate of approximately 55 beats/min and virtually absent FHR variability (second half of tracing, with scalp electrode). There were serious cardiac structural defects, and the child died shortly after birth. An alternative to doubling may be that the Doppler transducer was detecting atrial rather than ventricular activity. This may explain why there appears to be FHR variability in the first half of the tracing.

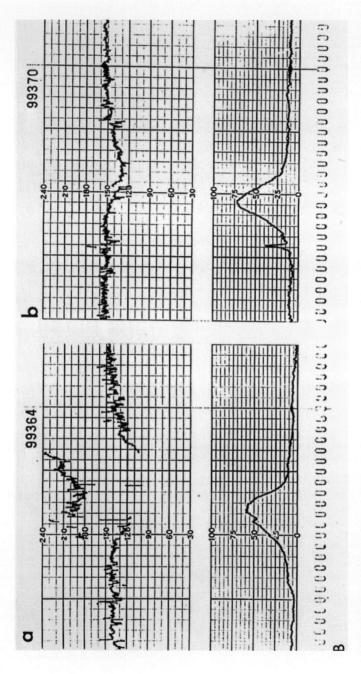

**FIGURE 7–11.**    A. Doubling of the heart rate during a deceleration B. This phenomenon has obscured the true nature of the late deceleration which was recorded accurately 24 minutes later.

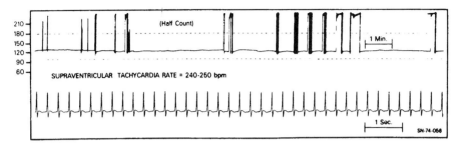

**FIGURE 7–12.** Halving of the FHR at high rates because of the limited ability of the machine to follow rates above 240 beats/min. (Courtesy of Schifrin BS. Workbook in Fetal Heart Rate Monitoring.)

## II UTERINE ACTIVITY

### A Intraamniotic Catheter

The internal, invasive method of detecting uterine activity consists of placement of a soft plastic open-ended or transducer-tipped catheter transcervically into the amniotic cavity (Fig. 7–17). These catheters detect pressure changes by means of a strain gauge transducer. These pressure changes are translated to an electrical signal, which is displayed and calibrated directly in millimeters of mercury of pressure.

Insertion of the catheter is facilitated by the use of a rigid plastic introducer, through which the flexible intraamniotic catheter is threaded. The introducer (with its catheter inside) is placed at the edge of the cervix between one's fingers, either lateral or posterior to the fetus. The introducer should not be advanced farther, because uterine perforation could occur. The flexible catheter then is threaded into the amniotic cavity until a marker point (generally at 25 to 45 cm) is at the labia. Should resistance be noted or should the catheter curl back toward the labia, a different point of insertion is selected.

Calibration for "zero" pressure varies depending on the type of intraamniotic catheter used, and whether the transducer is at the catheter tip or external to the uterus. A popular current version has one lumen for pressure measurement, and a second open-ended lumen for fluid administration for amnioinfusion (see Chapter 8).

### B Tokodynamometer

The tokodynamometer (*tokos* is Greek for childbirth) is an external device that is strapped to the maternal abdominal wall, generally over the uterine fundus. The tightening of the fundus with each contraction is detected by pressure on

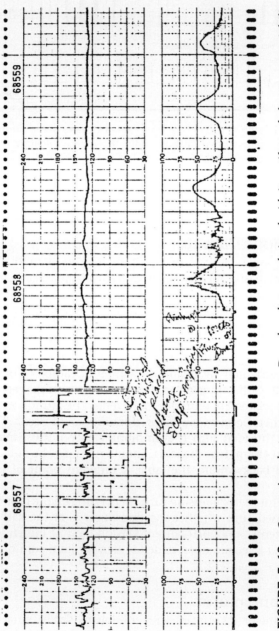

**FIGURE 7–13.** Comparison between a poor Doppler ultrasound signal with its artifactual short-term variability and the more accurate signal from the direct ECG electrode. The absent variability was obscured in the Doppler mode.

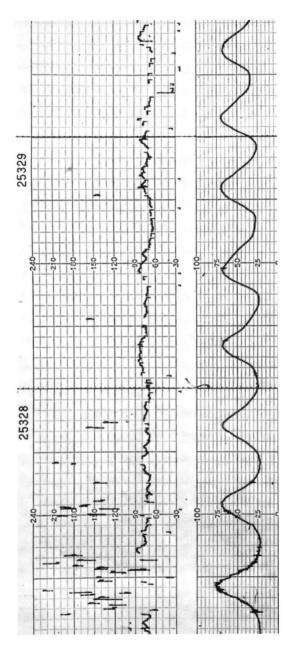

**FIGURE 7–14.**   Maternal heart rate recorded in the presence of a dead fetus following abruptio placentae. The apparently good long-term variability is inconsistent with this degree and duration of bradycardia. The frequent contractions and unrelaxing uterine activity also are typical of an abruption, because blood extravasates into the myometrium to set up multiple foci of irritation.

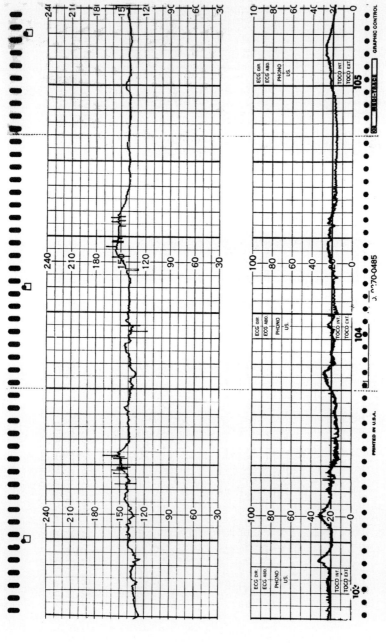

**FIGURE 7–15.** Note the apparently normal FHR variability in the first half of the tracing, at a paper speed of 1 cm/min. There is clearly decreased variability in the second half of the tracing, with a paper speed of 3 cm/min. Because an important aspect of FHR interpretation is pattern recognition, it is strongly recommended that a standard speed of 3 cm/min be used. (Courtesy of Dr. B. Block.)

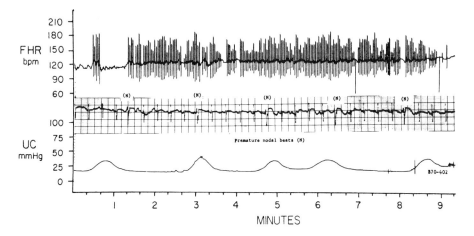

**FIGURE 7–16.** Arrhythmias appear as bizarre changes with a certain amount of regularity to them. Contrast this phenomenon with the irregular artifact in Figure 7–8. For example, an asystole is a rapid drop of the pen to half of the adjacent rates for a single heart beat. A premature ventricular contraction has a sudden increase in rate (commonly 10 or 20 beats/min) and an immediate decrease in rate, each for one beat, because of the shorter interval to the ventricular complex and the longer interval, which includes the compensatory pause. (Courtesy of Schifrin BS. Workbook in Fetal Heart Rate Monitoring.)

a small button in the center of the transducer, and uterine activity is displayed on the recorder. In a sense the apparatus acts just like the hand on the abdomen, detecting uterine activity. The tokodynamometer detects frequency and often duration of uterine contractions but ordinarily cannot be

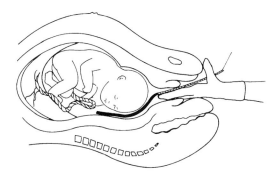

**FIGURE 7–17.** The technique of placing the intraamniotic catheter transcervically. Note that the rigid plastic introducer is guarded by the fingertips to prevent accidental perforation of the uterus.

calibrated for intensity as in direct pressure measurements. Use of the experienced hand for determining intensity of a contraction may be more accurate than this device. A research modification uses a circumferential ring that allows its attachment with a standard tension, so that it can be at least partially calibrated for pressure.

A potential additional disadvantage of the external device results from the fact that it works best with the woman in the supine position and with minimal maternal movement. This requirement may not be optimal for maternal comfort, fetal well-being, or progress in labor (see Chapter 15). In addition, some women find the belt confining and the tokodynamometer button uncomfortable.

## REFERENCES

1. Boehm FH, Fields LM, Hutchison JM, et al. The indirectly obtained fetal heart rate: Comparison of first- and second-generation electronic fetal monitors. Am J Obstet Gynecol 1986; 155:10–14.

2. Divon MY, Torres FP, Yeh S-Y, Paul RH. Autocorrelation techniques in fetal monitoring. Am J Obstet Gynecol 1985; 151:2–6.

3. Hon EH. An Atlas of Fetal Heart Rate Patterns. Harty Press, New Haven, CT, 1968.

4. Morgenstern J. Fetal monitor test—a brief summary. Application note, Hewlett Packard. Based on: Morgenstern J, Abels T, Hollbrügge P, et al. CTG-Geräte Test '93, Hrsg: Medizinische Einrichtungen der Heinrich-Heine-Universität, Frauenklinik, Düsseldorf, 1994/95.

# Chapter Eight

# Ancillary Methods and In Utero Treatment

In order to understand the role of ancillary testing in fetal heart rate (FHR) evaluation, an historical perspective is necessary.

Fetal blood sampling (FBS) was introduced in the early 1960s by Erich Saling of Berlin as a primary means of evaluating the fetus during labor.[23, 24] At approximately the same time, continuous beat-to-beat FHR monitoring during labor was being evaluated by Hon[12] and by Caldeyro-Barcia and coworkers.[6] From these two forms of intrapartum surveillance a combined system evolved, which included FHR screening during labor and the use of blood sampling in certain selected cases, indicated by potentially or actually "ominous" FHR patterns.[31] Subsequently, both retrospective and prospective studies showed that much simpler tests, the scalp stimulation test, or vibroacoustic stimulation, could give information equally reliable to that of FBS in many cases.

These techniques will be discussed here, together with their validation, limitations, and acceptance into current intrapartum management. Stimulation testing continues to gain widespread acceptance, while FBS has decreasing popularity,[8, 11, 20] so these techniques will be described in this order. In addition, in utero treatment of the fetus to attempt to optimize respiratory gas exchange will also be discussed.

---

 FETAL STIMULATION TESTING

## A Scalp Stimulation

During studies involving FBS in a research protocol Miller and his colleagues noted a high correlation between the occurrence of accelerations of the FHR

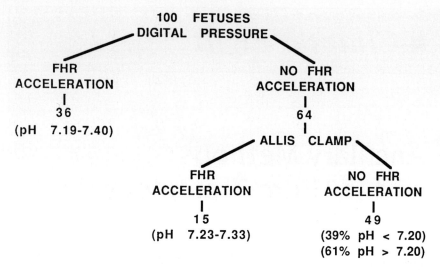

**FIGURE 8–1.** Results of a prospective trial of the scalp stimulation test, showing relationship between fetal blood pH and acceleration with digital stimulation or stimulation with an Allis clamp applied to the scalp in 100 fetuses. (Modified from Clark SL, Gimovsky ML, Miller FC. The scalp stimulation test: A clinical alternative to fetal scalp blood sampling. Am J Obstet Gynecol 1984; 148:274–277.)

during scalp puncture for obtaining a blood sample, and a "normal" pH value (i.e., above 7.20). In a subsequent prospective trial this observation was validated, and hence began its introduction into clinical practice.[7]

The technique is exceedingly simple. In the case of suspected fetal acidosis the scalp is digitally stimulated during vaginal examination and the FHR monitor observed for an acceleration of 15 seconds duration, peaking 15 beats/min above the baseline FHR. Should this maneuver fail to elicit an acceleration, the original workers closed an Allis clamp on the scalp, though few clinicians now resort to this. The results of the trial are summarized in Figure 8–1. Approximately 50 percent of the babies accelerated, and had normal pH. Of those that did not, approximately 60 percent had a normal pH, and the remainder were acidotic. Thus at least 50 percent were saved the necessity of a FBS.

A potential limitation of this result is that the number of fetuses responding with an acceleration is likely to be variable depending on the pattern prompting the test. Thus, if one uses fetal stimulation whenever there are mild variable decelerations in the presence of normal FHR variability, then positive results will be high. However, if one reserves the test for cases where there is reduced or absent variability in the presence of variable or late decelerations, then the success rate will be lower.

## B  Vibroacoustic Stimulation

This test was borrowed directly from its usage in antepartum monitoring, and the technique is described in Chapter 2.

The test depends on the provocation of an acceleration of the FHR following a 1-second transabdominal vibroacoustic stimulation over the region of the fetal vertex. The significance of a positive test is the same as that of a positive scalp stimulation test.[25]

The limitations and success appear to be similar to that described above for the scalp stimulation test. Thus the success rate is likely to be higher if it is applied in the case of relatively benign FHR patterns.

## FETAL BLOOD SAMPLING

## A  Instrumentation

The equipment used for collecting fetal blood anaerobically is sold in kit form. It consists of (1) an endoscope, (2) a light source, (3) a blade and blade holder, (4) sponges and holder, (5) capillary tubing, preheparinized, (6) ethyl chloride, and (7) silicone grease.

The machinery for determining pH and carbon dioxide tension in the blood is more complex. A number of blood gas analyzers are available commercially, most of which are automated, and all work on the same general principle. One measures the pH on anaerobic blood samples by transferring blood from the capillary tube to a glass electrode, suitably calibrated, and keeping it at 37° C. The reproducibility of measurements and the variation among even well-calibrated machines are of the order of 0.03 pH units.[30]

Carbon dioxide tension is measured on the same machine but with a separately calibrated carbon dioxide tension electrode. This technique also operates on the glass electrode principle. Generally, 0.25 ml (the capacity of the glass capillary collection tube) will suffice for measurement of both pH and carbon dioxide tension. In current blood gas machines oxygen tension is simultaneously measured.

Warm-up and calibration time on this equipment takes a minimum of 30 minutes, so in order to be practical the machine must be left on continuously if it is to be used in obstetric management. Such devices are generally available in neonatal intensive care units (NICUs) 24 hours a day, where technicians who are expert in the calibration and maintenance of this equipment are present. For hospitals without NICUs, the chance of being able to obtain accurate, rapid micro-blood gas analysis is unpredictable, because central clinical laboratories may be unfamiliar with microsamples, and turn-around time is unacceptably long. In some institutions dedicated blood gas machines are available in labor and delivery units. However, the need for quality control, maintenance, and accuracy generally makes this impractical. There is a commercially available pH meter, which is simpler to maintain, but this gives incomplete information.

## B  Technique of Fetal Blood Collection

Fetal blood is sampled by stabbing the fetal presenting part with a small blade, approximately 2 mm wide and 1.5 mm long. The resulting droplet of blood is collected in a glass capillary tube, approximately 30 cm long, which has been pretreated with heparin. Access to the fetus is facilitated by means of a cone-shaped endoscope with a light source, placed through the vagina against the fetus. The endoscope also permits cleansing of the sampling site with a sponge and exclusion of amniotic fluid and blood (Fig. 8–2).

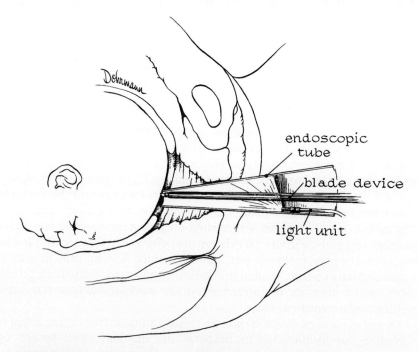

**FIGURE 8–2.** Technique of obtaining fetal blood from scalp during labor. (From Creasy RK, Parer JT. Prenatal care and diagnosis. In Rudolph AM, ed. Pediatrics, 16th ed. Appleton-Century-Crofts, New York, 1977, p. 121. Used by permission.)

Reactive hyperemia of fetal skin may be produced by spraying with ethyl chloride. Containment of the blood droplet can be aided by use of a smear of silicone cream on the fetal skin. This technique is similar to that of the adult "finger stick" for obtaining small quantities of blood, but it is important in the fetus to obtain free-flowing blood and to collect it from the center of the droplet, protecting it from air as much as possible. Generally, a single stab will suffice, but on occasion an X-shaped incision is necessary. If fetal hair is copious, it can be brushed aside or trimmed. Sampling should be done over the scalp or buttock and not on the brow, face, or genitals.

The capillary tube contains approximately 0.25 ml of blood, which is sufficient for measurement of pH and carbon dioxide tension in current micro-blood gas analysis machines. It is our practice to obtain two specimens, so that duplicate analyses can be made.

After collection of the blood, a sponge is pressed against the sampling site until hemostasis is evident during contractions. There is no theoretical limit to the number of samples that can be taken, although, as a practical matter, numerous samples (e.g., greater than 10) can result in widespread soft tissue trauma to the fetus.

## C Validation of the Technique

Several approaches to the question of validation have been taken. It has been shown in fetal monkeys that the values in blood obtained from the scalp are closely related to simultaneously sampled blood from the carotid artery and the jugular vein. In fact, the pH generally falls between the values from these vessels. In 5 percent of cases, the pH of capillary blood was found to be more than 0.1 unit lower than that of carotid arterial blood. In human newborns, a good correlation has been demonstrated between scalp blood pH taken shortly before delivery and umbilical cord samples.[3]

Further validation of the technique is seen in correlations between scalp blood pH and newborn outcome.[2] This is illustrated in Figure 8–3, in which the Apgar score at 2 minutes is related to scalp blood pH collected shortly before delivery. In this investigation, a blood pH above 7.25 at this time was associated with 2-minute Apgar score of greater than 7 in 92 percent of infants. A pH of less than 7.15 was associated with a score of less than 6 in 80 percent of cases. A pH between 7.15 and 7.25 in the second stage of labor was unreliable for predicting the condition of the baby at birth by 2-minute Apgar score in 47 percent of cases. No better correlation was found between Apgar score and base deficit differences ($\Delta BD$) between maternal and fetal blood, although fetuses with a low pH and a small $\Delta BD$ were more likely to be acidotic because of equilibration with fixed acids from the mother. This finding is of less concern than the situation in which fetuses are acidotic because of their own necessity for anaerobic metabolism and, hence, lactate production. In

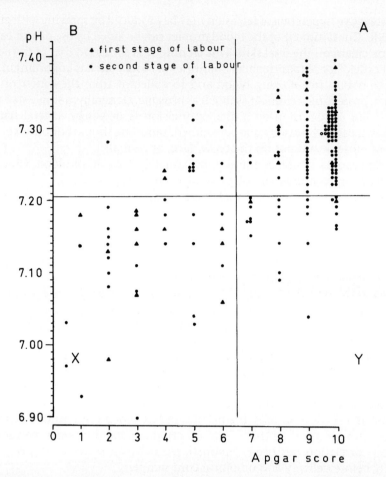

**FIGURE 8–3.** Relationship between fetal blood pH and Apgar score at 2 minutes. All samples were taken shortly before delivery. The arbitrary lines separate fetuses regarded as vigorous (Apgar score 7 or above) and those with "normal" pH (above 7.2). Note that there is a general relationship between the two variables (segments A and X) and also approximately 30 percent spillover into the false-normal and false-abnormal groups (B and Y). (From Beard RW, Morris ED, Clayton SG. pH of foetal capillary blood as an indicator of the condition of the foetus. J Obstet Gynaecol Br Commonw 1967; 74:812–822. Used by permission.)

fact, babies who are acidotic because of equilibration of fixed acids with the mother generally are vigorous at birth. Other investigators similarly have found a correlation between fetal blood pH and Apgar score.[27]

Another approach to validation has been to relate fetal blood pH to "abnormal" FHR patterns.[13, 17] Unfortunately, such an approach is not strictly valid, because the former observation is used to substantiate the latter. Nevertheless, some impressive correlations have been noted (Table 8–1). This landmark report was felt by many to confirm the ominousness of certain FHR patterns. Of great importance, however, is a reanalysis of these data in a study published 6 years later.[21] Instead of continuum of acidosis in the various groups of FHR patterns seen in Table 8–1, these investigators showed that they could separate patients with late decelerations into two distinct groups based on the degree of FHR variability (Fig. 8–4). Those with average or higher variability were significantly less acidotic than those with decreased variability. In fact, in the presence of mild or moderate late decelerations with average variability, the average baby was not acidotic.

This surprising finding is explained by the presence of two distinct classes of late decelerations, those resulting from neurogenic (vagal) reflexes and those caused by hypoxic myocardial depression or failure (see Chapter 9). FBS can help to distinguish the two etiologies, but the presence of FHR variability and stimulation tests are a more convenient means to accomplish this objective.

In summary, FBS is a valid technique for determining fetal acid-base status. The fetal acid-base status relates to fetal outcome (by Apgar score) with an accuracy of 80 to 90 percent, at best, and is correlated with FHR patterns and their presumed reflection of asphyxia, although there are many important exceptions. The current place of FBS in intrapartum management will be described below.

---

##  IN UTERO TREATMENT

### A  Conservative and Simple Techniques

It is now well recognized that in certain cases fetal oxygenation can be improved, acidosis relieved, and variant FHR patterns modified or abolished

**TABLE 8–1.  Relationship Between Fetal Blood pH and Fetal Heart Rate Patterns in Preceding 20 Minutes**

| FHR *Deceleration* Pattern | Fetal Blood pH[a] |
|---|---|
| Early, mild variable, or absent | $7.30 \pm 0.04$ |
| Moderate variable | $7.26 \pm 0.04$ |
| Mild or moderate late | $7.22 \pm 0.06$ |
| Severe late or variable | $7.14 \pm 0.07$ |

[a]Approximate mean ± standard deviation.

Modified from Kubli et al. Observations on heart rate and pH in the human fetus during labor. Am J Obstet Gynecol 1969; 104:1190–1206.

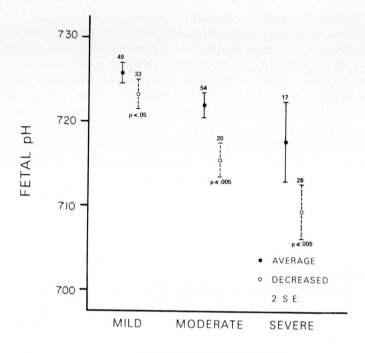

LATE DECELERATION

**FIGURE 8–4.** Relationship between fetal blood pH and severity of late decelerations at time of blood sampling. Each FHR classification is further divided into average (greater than 5 beats/min) or decreased (less than 5 beats/min) FHR variability. (From Paul RH, Suidan AK, Yeh SY, et al. Clinical fetal monitoring: VII. The evaluation and significance of intrapartum baseline FHR variability. Am J Obstet Gynecol 1975; 123:206–210. Used by permission.)

by certain modes of treatment. The events that result in interference with placental exchange (recognized by certain FHR patterns) are presented in Table 8–2, together with the recommended treatment maneuvers and presumed mechanisms for improving fetal oxygenation.

These should be the primary maneuvers carried out, and if the potential asphyxial insult is acute and reversible and the fetus was previously normoxic, there is an excellent chance that the variant FHR pattern will be abolished. If the variant pattern is late decelerations, they are most likely of the reflex type, rather than those caused by myocardial failure. The

**TABLE 8–2.  Intrauterine Treatment for Variant Fetal Heart Rate Patterns**

| Causes | Possible Resulting FHR Patterns | Corrective Maneuver | Mechanism |
|---|---|---|---|
| Hypotension (e.g., supine hypotension, conduction anesthesia) | Bradycardia, late decelerations | Intravenous fluids Position change Ephedrine | Return of uterine blood flow toward normal |
| Excessive uterine activity | Bradycardia, late decelerations | Decrease in oxytocin Lateral position | Same as above |
| Transient umbilical cord compression | Variable decelerations | Change in maternal position (e.g., left or right lateral, or Trendelenburg) Amnioinfusion | Return of umbilical blood flow toward normal by decreasing cord compression "Pads" the cord, protecting it from compression |
| Head compression, usually second stage | Variable decelerations | Push only with alternate contractions | Return of umbilical blood flow toward normal |
| Decreased uterine blood flow during uterine contraction below limits of fetal basal oxygen needs | Late decelerations | Change in maternal position (e.g., left or right lateral, or Trendelenburg) Establishment of maternal hyperoxia Tocolytic agents (e.g., terbutaline) | Enhancement of uterine blood flow (UBF) toward optimum Increase in maternal-fetal oxygen gradient Decrease in contractions or uterine tonus, thus reducing associated decrease in UBF |

*Table continued on following page*

**TABLE 8–2.  Intrauterine Treatment for Variant Fetal Heart Rate Patterns** (*Continued*)

| Causes | Possible Resulting FHR Patterns | Corrective Maneuver | Mechanism |
|---|---|---|---|
| Prolonged asphyxia | Decreasing FHR variability in appropriate setting[a] | Change in maternal position (e.g., left or right lateral, or Trendelenburg) Establishment of maternal hyperoxia Tocolytic agents (e.g., terbutaline) | Enhancement of UBF toward optimum Increase in maternal–fetal oxygen gradient Decrease in contractions or uterine tonus, thus reducing associated decrease in UBF |

[a]NB: During labor this is virtually always preceded by a heart rate pattern signifying asphyxial stress (e.g., late decelerations (usually severe), severe variable decelerations, or a prolonged bradycardia). This is not necessarily so in the antepartum period, before the onset of uterine contractions.

presumption is that the oxygen deficit is relatively small, and maneuvers such as those in Table 8–2 make up the deficiency. For example, fetal oxygen tension increased by 5 mmHg during maternal hyperoxia, when the mother's oxygen tension rose to 300 mmHg.[15] This fetal oxygen tension increment represents 2 ml $O_2 \cdot dl^{-1}$ in fetal blood oxygen content on the steep part of the oxygen dissociation curve (see Fig. 3–7).

During labor an FHR pattern with decreasing variability due to asphyxia is virtually always preceded by a heart rate pattern signifying asphyxial stress [e.g., late decelerations, variable decelerations (usually severe), or a prolonged bradycardia]. In the antepartum period, however, before the onset of uterine contractions, this does not necessarily hold, and a fetus may develop decreasing or absent variability due to asphyxia without periodic or baseline FHR changes. In addition, there is some evidence that the normal evolution to decreased or absent variability sometimes occurs with relatively minor decelerations in cases of chorioamnionitis, and dysmaturity.

If the FHR patterns cannot be improved (i.e., if the stress patterns indicative of peripheral tissue or central tissue asphyxia persist for a significant period), further diagnosis (by ancillary techniques) or delivery may be indicated.

Certain patterns are of such a severe character that immediate delivery without ancillary testing, such as fetal scalp sampling, is warranted if they cannot rapidly be relieved. They include patterns with a smooth baseline and severe, uncorrectable late or variable decelerations, or a prolonged bradycardia below 60 beats/min with a smooth baseline. It is reasonable to assume that such fetuses are either already asphyxiated or will soon become so, and to carry out rapid delivery.

# B  Amnioinfusion

The theory of variable decelerations being caused by cord compression has given rise to the technique of amnioinfusion.[19] In this straightforward technique sterile crystalloid is infused into the amniotic cavity through an intrauterine catheter, with an initial bolus of 250 to 1000 ml and a maintenance of about 2 to 3 ml/mm (Fig. 8–5). This has been shown to result in a lowered incidence of severe variable decelerations and may allow a vaginal delivery instead of a cesarean section for presumed fetal asphyxia.[26] It may also decrease the incidence of meconium aspiration when the meconium is thick.[10, 28] It appears to be more efficacious in premature fetuses than term fetuses, and is not so effective in the second stage of labor, lending support to the theory that second-stage variable decelerations are due to head and not cord compression.

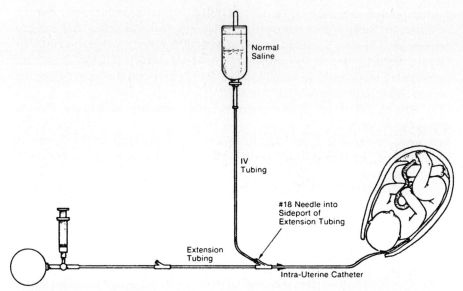

**FIGURE 8–5.** The original technique used for amnioinfusion. More recent catheters have a double lumen so that the pressure is measured through one and a separate port allows amnioinfusion. (From Miyazaki FS, Taylor NA. Saline amnioinfusion for relief of variable or prolonged decelerations. Am J Obstet Gynecol 1983; 146:670–677. Used by permission.)

---

# IV FETAL HEART RATE PATTERN MANAGEMENT AND THE ROLE OF ANCILLARY TESTING AND TECHNIQUES

Rational management of labor with the use of continuous FHR monitoring requires an understanding of the following four topics:

1. The recognition, clinical significance, and limitations of measurement of FHR variability (see Chapter 9).

2. The spectrum of asphyxia [i.e., the continuum from mild asphyxia to severe, fatal degrees, and the physiologic compensations available to the fetus in the earlier phases (see Chapters 4, 5 and 10)].

3. The influence of in utero treatment of the fetus, and its presumed role in improving fetal oxygenation and modifying or preventing fetal asphyxial stress, as recognized in certain FHR patterns.

4. The indications for ancillary testing based on the findings in FHR screening, and an understanding of the limitations and complications of

interpretation of stimulation testing and fetal acid-base status, and the evolution of FHR patterns with decreasing or increasing oxygenation.

The final topic will be described here. The incorporation of ancillary testing into a system of obstetric management based on FHR screening has been described previously by others.[1, 7, 25, 27, 32] The approach that will be discussed here is somewhat different, in that it relies heavily on the high prognostic accuracy of FHR variability in predicting a vigorous fetus, even in certain cases of peripheral blood acidemia.[4, 16, 20]

## A  Indications for Ancillary Testing

Fetal stimulation testing or FBS may be beneficial for patient management in the following situations:

1. Absent FHR variability on initial application of the monitor in the absence of a clear cause [e.g., recent large maternal dose of centrally depressing drugs (see Chapter 12)].
2. Absent FHR variability in the case of a fetus with potential asphyxia, even in the presence of centrally depressing drugs (e.g., a gravida undergoing magnesium sulfate treatment for pre-eclampsia).
3. Late decelerations with decreasing variability and a pattern that cannot be abolished in a reasonable time (e.g., 30 minutes).
4. Variable decelerations with decreasing variability and a pattern that cannot be abolished in a reasonable time (e.g., 30 minutes).
5. Puzzling, or unusual, unexplained patterns (e.g., an intermittent sinusoidal or a regular "picket fence" pattern that may simulate variability, except for its repetitiousness).

Of lesser value is use of ancillary testing in the following situations:

1. Late decelerations that cannot be abolished in approximately 30 minutes, even in the presence of good variability. A knowledge that serious acidosis is absent may allow one to estimate the urgency of the situation.
2. Severe variable decelerations with normal baseline variability that cannot be relieved in a reasonable time (30 minutes). This indication has limited usefulness, because the fetus has a very high likelihood of being vigorous despite the pH value, provided variability is retained. If FBS is used, timing of sampling is important, because substantial respiratory acidosis can develop during the deceleration but is relieved afterward; therefore, one must obtain sufficient blood to measure the carbon dioxide tension and to calculate the base excess.

Fetal ancillary testing has not been found useful in the presence of normal FHR patterns, despite potentially hazardous clinical situations, such as in cases of thick meconium or diabetes mellitus. Its use following resolution of late, variable, or prolonged decelerations also has potential problems, such as false-abnormal stimulation tests, or in the case of FBS sometimes the acidosis is resolving, and abnormal values must be followed serially until they become normal. A preferable approach is to follow the heart rate pattern to normality and to manage solely on the basis of it.

If a vigorous newborn with a high Apgar score (greater than 7 at 5 minutes) is the ultimate objective, it is important to examine how accurately this outcome is predicted by either the fetal pH or the FHR. The presence of normal FHR variability predicts a vigorous fetus in more than 97 percent of cases.[4, 16] In contrast, a normal fetal pH predicts a vigorous fetus in 90 percent of cases,[2] and a low pH predicts a depressed fetus with only 80 percent reliability (Fig. 8.3). In view of the high prognostic reliability of normal FHR variability, there seems little point in taking pH samples of such a fetus, because the infant will likely be vigorous regardless of the pH value obtained. Similarly, fetal stimulation testing has a false abnormal rate, so should not be fully relied upon to imply fetal compromise in the face of an otherwise normal FHR pattern.

Fetal blood sampling also is not useful in the presence of certain unrelieved sinister FHR patterns (e.g., absent FHR variability with severe and worsening periodic patterns). These fetuses either are already, or will likely soon become, asphyxiated, and rapid delivery is preferable to taking the time for FBS. However stimulation testing is probably worthwhile in such situations, because of its rapid performance, but unless the response to stimulation is dramatic, one still has to make the clinical decision whether to act on the original tracing, or to alter the presumed diagnosis of actual or impending asphyxia based on the provoked acceleration. In addition to this group, many authorities also would include the aforementioned categories 3 and 4, in which there is decreasing FHR variability in the presence of a stress pattern, in the category of FBS having limited usefulness, although stimulation testing once again can be useful.

# B Limitation of Fetal Blood Sampling

## CONTRAINDICATIONS
Fetal blood sampling should not be performed when the fetus has a known or a suspected blood dyscrasia (e.g., hemophilia or von Willebrand's disease). Fetal deaths resulting from excessive blood loss have been reported in such cases.

Fetal blood sampling can be performed only after rupture of the membranes, so any contraindications to this procedure also apply to FBS. A further contraindication is the likelihood of multiple sampling; that is, in the case of a patient early in a predicted long labor with an FHR pattern requiring frequent sampling (e.g., over a 6-hour active phase with samples required every 30 minutes). After this many samples (namely, 12), the soft tissue damage to the fetal scalp can be considerable, and cesarean section may be deemed preferable. In addition, the procedure may interfere with the labor process because of the necessity for positioning the mother (e.g., in lithotomy) to obtain samples. Also of great importance is the discomfort caused to the mother by multiple sampling.

A potential disadvantage occurs with the use of the vacuum extractor after FBS. Although employment of this device is not absolutely contraindicated, one must be wary of using it on a fetus whose scalp has had numerous punctures for FBS.

FBS, and also the use of a fetal scalp electrode, is relatively contraindicated in the presence of a number of maternal infectious diseases, namely human immunodeficiency virus, herpes, and hepatitis. Amnionitis is considered a relative contraindication because of the possibility of increasing the risk of fetal scalp infection.

## COMPLICATIONS OF FETAL BLOOD SAMPLING

Fetal death caused by exsanguination has been reported in the presence of unsuspected fetal coagulopathy. In addition, there have been cases of neonatal bleeding resulting from resolution of scalp vasoconstriction that previously had prevented bleeding.

The incidence of scalp infections has been cited as less than 1 percent, with the large majority of newborns requiring only local treatment (e.g., hair trimming, disinfection). With today's more common use of FHR monitoring with spiral electrodes, the incidence of complications is somewhat unclear, because FHR monitoring always precedes FBS. The infectious and other complications of FHR monitoring are discussed in Chapter 15.

In summary, if mortality resulting from coagulopathies is excluded, the infectious complications of FBS are quantitatively minor and are of less importance than is the potentially irreversible problem of asphyxial brain damage, which FBS may assist in avoiding.

## EFFECT ON CESAREAN SECTION

Some randomized and nonrandomized trials of the efficacy of intrapartum FHR monitoring have shown that the cesarean section rate tends to be higher if FBS is not used (see Chapter 15). There is no similar randomized trial with stimulation testing. There is no consensus in reports regarding the extent of this finding, but the cesarean section rate undoubtedly depends on the method of interpretation of FHR patterns and, particularly, on the degree to which one depends on FHR baseline variability. It has been implied that use of a means of interpretation of FHR based primarily on the presence of variability and accelerations will lead to very few cases of unnecessary cesarean section,[11] although this hypothesis has not yet been proven unequivocally.

## INTERPRETATION OF RESULTS OF FBS

A commonly heard maxim is that if pH is above 7.20, the fetus is normal, and if pH is below 7.20, the fetus is abnormal, and delivery by the most expeditious route is indicated. This approach, however, is somewhat simplistic.

A more appropriate, although still unsatisfactory, belief is that values above 7.25 are normal, and values below 7.20 are abnormal (see Chapter 6). Values between 7.20 and 7.25 need to be interpreted on the basis of many other important factors, which will be discussed in the following sections.

***Maternal pH and Base Excess*** It is hoped that, in FBS, values of pH and base excess mirror the fetal dependence on anaerobic metabolism and, of lesser importance, on carbon dioxide retention. In some cases, however, maternal metabolic acidosis is present, and over a period of time there is equilibration of the fixed acids across the placenta. This situation occurs most commonly in a prolonged stressful labor, in which there is maternal volume depletion and probable peripheral vasoconstriction with partial dependence on anaerobic metabolism, possibly accompanied by a mild starvation ketosis. In such cases, maternal arterial pH may approach 7.30, and base excess approximately $-8$Eq $\cdot$ L$^{-1}$. This degree of maternal acidosis is generally not hazardous, and it is asymptomatic and unrecognized unless deliberately measured. It may, however, result in fetal acidosis, with the pH often below 7.20, which, in fact, mirrors the maternal state and is not an indication of intrinsic fetal dependence on anaerobic metabolism.

When an unexpectedly low fetal pH is obtained, it is recommended that maternal acid-base state be measured. This procedure is performed most conveniently by collecting a maternal venous specimen from a large vein (e.g., antecubital) into a heparinized syringe, without blood stasis. Thus, a tourniquet may be used for needle entry into the vein, but it should be removed before collection of the blood to avoid causing local tissue acidosis. Should doubt arise regarding the validity of the samples, a maternal arterial sample may be drawn.

Interpretation of base excess differences ($\Delta$BE) between maternal and fetal blood has been attempted, generally without great success on a quantitative level.[2] A fetal blood base excess of less than $-10$ mEq $\cdot$ L$^{-1}$ should be viewed with caution, because this finding suggests a $\Delta$BE of more than $-6$ mEq $\cdot$ L$^{-1}$.

***Accuracy of Sampling*** Fetal blood samples from the fetal caput succedaneum may be diluted by tissue fluid and may reflect local scalp stasis, so the values obtained may be erroneously low. Saling[23] maintains that this situation is rare, occurring only 3 percent of the time.

A further source of error may be contamination of the specimen with air during collection. This phenomenon will be observed as breaks in the column of blood and generally will result in an increased oxygen tension, a decreased carbon dioxide tension, and an artificially elevated pH. Machine calibration is important and generally must be accepted on faith. Wood, in a comprehensive discussion of errors, has stated that a change in scalp pH can be considered relevant only when it is more than 0.05 pH unit.[30]

***Type of Acidosis*** Given a pH below 7.20, metabolic acidosis (e.g., a base excess of −12 mEq · L$^{-1}$) is of more concern than is a respiratory acidosis (e.g., a carbon dioxide tension of 70 mmHg) because of the ease with which carbon dioxide can be removed, and because the former finding implies fetal dependence on anaerobic metabolism. Hence, it is important to measure the carbon dioxide tension (and to calculate the base excess) each time one obtains an abnormal or borderline pH value.

***Stage of Labor*** A number of methods have been suggested for the management of labor using FBS. These methods have been based on absolute values of pH and on rates of change of pH.[23] Such algorithms are of merit as a basis for discussion, but lose their value when applied to individual cases. The inadequacy is exemplified when one considers the stage of labor: a borderline pH of 7.18, with a base excess of −10 mEq · L$^{-1}$, would be of greater significance in the early active phase of the labor of a primigravida than in the late active phase of the labor of a multipara.

***Transient Versus Permanent Insult*** Fetal acidosis may be seen with late or variable decelerations and may even be apparent some time after correction of these patterns. Acidosis also is seen (1) with maternal hypotension (caused by sympathetic blockade following regional anesthesia or the supine hypotensive syndrome), (2) following hyperstimulation with oxytocin, or (3) following a maternal seizure. All of these examples are episodes of transient reduction in exchange of the respiratory gases, which generally can be corrected. Hence, if they are corrected, and if the FHR pattern returns to normal, pH determinations are not indicated and, in fact, may be detrimental (albeit primarily from a financial standpoint), because if acidosis is present, multiple determinations may be necessary until the acidosis resolves.

In contrast, a permanent insult to the placental oxygen transfer mechanism, by partial placental abruption or by progressive acidosis in labor in a gravida with severe preeclampsia and compromised placental function, may be expected to be irreversible, and patient management must be more aggressive in these cases.

***Influence of*** **In Utero** ***Treatment*** Fetal blood sampling should not be performed until after the aforementioned treatment maneuvers have been attempted (Table 8–2). If these measures fail to improve or correct the abnormality within a reasonable time (e.g., 15 minutes), then FBS should be used, if appropriate, according to the indications discussed earlier.

***Relationship in Time to Uterine Contractions***    It has been shown that
fetal pH tends to be lowest at the end of a variable deceleration and recovers
between contractions. This situation probably results from respiratory acidosis, but it can depress the pH profoundly. Furthermore, it has been shown that
the fetal oxygen tension falls during slowing of the heart rate by more than 15
beats/min with contractions. Hence, it is preferable to obtain the FBS just
before the next expected uterine contraction (Fig. 8–6), because it will best
reflect the baseline state of the fetus at this time.

***Relationship of pH to Fetal Heart Rate Pattern and Clinical Situa-
tion***    As with all laboratory tests in medicine, the pH of a fetal blood sample
must be interpreted with due regard to the whole clinical situation, including
the severity of any maternal illness, the likely conduct of labor, and the
accompanying FHR pattern. Thus, one would react more aggressively to a
borderline pH in a case of severe preeclampsia or maternal diabetes than in the
absence of these conditions. Also, in the presence of an FHR pattern of sinister
appearance (e.g., decreased or absent variability with intermittent smooth

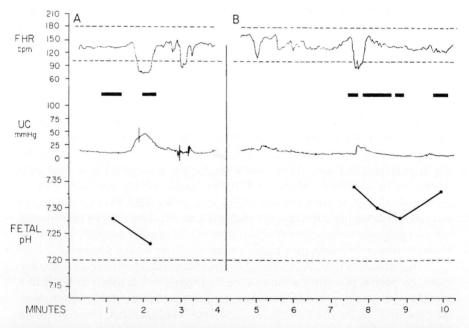

**FIGURE 8–6.**    Relationship of fetal blood pH to occurrence of variable decelerations.
The bars below the FHR tracing show the time over which blood was collected. Note that
pH is highest just before a deceleration and is lowest during or following it. This effect
occurs primarily because of retained carbon dioxide (i.e., respiratory acidosis). (From
Hon EH, Khazin AF. Biochemical studies of the fetus. I. The fetal pH measuring system.
Obstet Gynecol 1969; 33:219–236.)

periodic changes), one should be more intent on delivery when there is a borderline pH level.

***Practical Problems in Application of Fetal Blood Sampling*** Despite the hopes of investigators and proponents of FBS, the knowledge of this technique has diffused poorly from academic institutions to the community hospitals and nonuniversity institutions, where the vast majority of babies are delivered in the United States. There appear to be two reasons for this lack of knowledge: (1) the majority of people delivering babies were not trained in the technique or have not become sufficiently skilled for accurate use, and (2) relatively few institutions have microblood gas machines available 24 hours a day to give rapid, accurate results to the obstetric service.

One solution is to simplify the technique so that it can be applied as simply as FHR monitoring, by using a continuously recording pH electrode.[18] Such electrodes have been developed but have had major difficulties in clinical application. A more promising and potentially more practical device is the fetal pulse oximeter, which is currently undergoing clinical trials.[9]

The larger tertiary care institutions with NICUs already have blood gas machines with round-the-clock technicians who are skilled in handling small blood samples from premature infants. Many community hospitals, on the other hand, must depend on blood gas analysis from the central laboratory. The personnel in these facilities are accustomed to handling adult blood samples but rarely encounter the microsamples obtained from the fetus. In addition, the turn-around time from sampling to result may be too long for practical purposes.

Attempts have been made to place blood gas machines on the labor and delivery room floor, so that the blood samples may be analyzed by a house officer or an obstetrician. This practice has been of limited usefulness, primarily because the sophisticated machinery requires expert maintenance and calibration as well as experience in rectifying problems. It is not logical to hire three shifts of technicians daily to run the machine solely for obstetric purposes, because of the expense and infrequent use of the equipment.

A generous estimate of the use of FBS is in approximately 3 percent of patients in a mixed population. In a hospital delivering 2000 babies a year, or 6 per day, FBS would be used on an average once every 5 days. The expense of a machine solely for obstetric use therefore cannot be justified. The use of FBS will be even further decreased if the indications mentioned previously are taken into account. Acceptance of the aforementioned factors requires the acceptance of the high prognostic accuracy of normal FHR variability to predict a vigorous fetus, even in the presence of other FHR stress patterns. Only a small number of fetuses, probably less than 1 percent in most populations, have FHR patterns with absent or decreasing variability and with periodic changes that cannot be ascribed to drugs or other nonasphyxial causes. Part of this small group may unnecessarily go to cesarean section for fetal distress in the absence of FBS, but the influence of this technique on overall cesarean section rates will be minor.

***Summary of Fetal Blood Sampling***   In summary, a pH above 7.25 is normal and, depending on the severity of the FHR pattern, calls for repetition of testing at selected intervals of 20 to 60 minutes. A pH below 7.20, in the absence of maternal acidosis, calls for delivery within a reasonable period of time, generally less than 1 hour. The decision as to whether to deliver immediately (generally by cesarean section) or to temporize (e.g., to expect a vaginal delivery within this limited time) depends on the severity of the accompanying FHR pattern, the expected rapidity of delivery, and the severity of the maternal condition. Thus, one may temporize until a safe forceps delivery becomes possible.

There is no simple method for management of values between 7.20 and 7.25. These findings also must be interpreted with due regard for the severity of the FHR pattern, the likelihood of delivery within a reasonable time, the trend of the pH and base excess over a given period, the success of in utero treatment and so forth.

 ## UMBILICAL CORD BLOOD GASES AND ACID-BASE STATE

Although this is an intrapartum assessment technique, the results are not available until after delivery.

The technique is simple.[22] At the time of birth the cord is double clamped in two places about 25 cm apart. The cord is cut between each set of clamps, and blood is aspirated anaerobically from the umbilical artery and umbilical vein into heparinized syringes (Fig. 8–7). The bloods are then analyzed for pH and carbon dioxide and oxygen tension in the blood gas machine. As noted above the greatest accuracy is achieved with careful anaerobic collection, identification of umbilical artery (generally the smaller vessels) and vein (generally the larger and easier one), collection of sufficient volume (more than 0.5 ml) to minimize dilution and effects of inevitable air exposure, timely analysis (less than half an hour), and accurate recording.

It has been stated that the cord should be clamped immediately at birth, and before the first breath, to obtain the most representative in utero sample. While this is not particularly difficult if a baby is depressed, or at the time of cesarean section, there are some good reasons to delay clamping somewhat in the apparently normal, vigorous baby. In patient-oriented and natural-childbirth practices the newborn is usually given immediately to the mother and father, and not infrequently placed on the mother's abdomen. Immediate

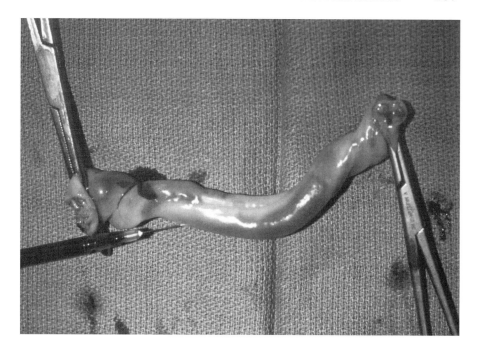

**FIGURE 8–7.** A double-clamped segment of umbilical cord immediately after birth. Blood has been aspirated from the umbilical artery, and blood is now being aspirated anaerobically from the larger umbilical vein.

clamping under these conditions will be intrusive, so we recommend clamping at a mutually opportune time.

The ideal time to clamp the cord is still controversial, with some advocates recommending that the attendant clamp immediately to prevent the transfusion of blood from the placenta, while others recommend waiting for the cord to stop pulsating, so that the newborn can obtain the "right amount" of blood. There is no good evidence for either of these extremes, and indeed nature has endowed the cord with a mechanism for spasm in mammalian species. Therefore we recommend an approach of moderation, with an intermediate time of clamping (e.g., about half a minute), unless, of course, there are other considerations such as resuscitation.

The effect of delaying clamping until after newborn breathing may be to alter the respiratory components of the blood gases (i.e., carbon dioxide and oxygen) rather than the metabolic components. The respiratory components are less important than the metabolic components. The importance of metabolic acidosis as an index of asphyxia is covered in Chapter 10, and normal values of umbilical cord blood gases are given in Chapter 6.

**TABLE 8–3. Blood Gas and Acid-Base State of Umbilical Cord Blood in the Case of a Cord Prolapse**

|  | Umbilical Artery | Umbilical Vein |
|---|---|---|
| pH | 7.03 | 7.35 |
| Carbon dioxide pressure (mm Hg) | 101 | 48 |
| Oxygen pressure (mm Hg) | 11 | 41 |
| Oxygen content (ml $O_2 \cdot dl^{-1}$) | 1.4 | 16.7 |
| Base excess (mEq $\cdot L^{-1}$) | −4 | +1 |

Modified from Riley WJ, Johnson JWC. Collecting and analyzing cord blood. Clin Obstet Gynecol 1993; 36:13–23.

The use of umbilical cord blood sampling appears to be increasing in clinical obstetrics for many reasons, not the least of which is for medicolegal purposes (see Chapter 16).

Our recommendation is to obtain cord blood gases at all deliveries, if logistically and financially feasible. If such a course is not possible, then we recommend they be obtained on all depressed (low Apgar score) babies, and those with an FHR pattern that suggests decompensation. Many clinicians would also recommend cord blood gases in such situations as cesarean section or operative vaginal delivery. If logistics or finances dictate only one specimen, then the umbilical artery is preferable, because it represents blood coming from the fetus, and there can be wide discrepancies between the values in the umbilical vein and artery under conditions of poor umbilical blood flow[5, 22] (Table 8–3).

An argument against obtaining only umbilical arterial blood has been raised by some who insist that one cannot always be sure that the specimen is not accidently venous unless both are obtained for comparison.[29] However, economic concerns may prevent adoption of this approach in North America.

A recent survey of university obstetricians in North America showed that the majority did obtain cord blood gases, at least selectively (e.g., with depressed babies or "abnormal" FHR trace), and at least from the umbilical artery. The majority also obtained the "full panel" rather than just pH.[14]

## REFERENCES

1. Beard RW, Filshie GM, Knight CA, Roberts GM. The significance of the changes in the continuous fetal heart rate in the first stage of labour. J Obstet Gynaecol Br Commonw 1971; 78:865–881.

2. Beard RW, Morris ED, Clayton SG. pH of foetal capillary blood as an indicator of the condition of the foetus. J Obstet Gynaecol Br Commonw 1967; 74:812–822.

3. Berg D, Saling E. The oxygen partial pressures in the human fetus during labor and delivery. In Longo LD, Bartels H, eds. Respiratory Gas Exchange and Blood Flow in the

Placenta. U.S. Department of Health, Education and Welfare Publications, Bethesda, MD, 1972, pp. 441–459.

4. Boehm FH. FHR variability: Key to fetal well-being. Contemp Obstet Gynecol: 1977; 9:57–65 .

5. Brar HS, Wong MK, Kirschbaum TH, Paul RH. Umbilical cord acid base changes associated with perinatal cardiac failure. Am J Obstet Gynecol 1988; 158:511–518.

6. Caldeyro-Barcia, R, Mendez-Bauer C, Poseiro JJ, et al. Control of human fetal heart rate during labor. In Cassels DE, ed. The Heart and Circulation in the Newborn and Infant. Grune & Stratton, New York, 1966, pp. 7–36.

7. Clark SL, Gimovsky ML, Miller FC. The scalp stimulation test: A clinical alternative to fetal scalp blood sampling. Am J Obstet Gynecol 1984; 148:274–277.

8. Clark SL, Paul RM. Intrapartum fetal surveillance: The role of fetal scalp blood sampling. Am J Obstet Gynecol 1985; 153:717–720.

9. Dildy GA, van den Berg PP, Katz M, Clark SL, Jongsma HW, Nijhuis JG, Loucks CA. Intrapartum fetal pulse oximetry: Fetal oxygen saturation trends during labor and relation to delivery outcome. Am J Obstet Gynecol 1994; 171:679–684.

10. Dye T, Aubry R, Gross S, Artal R. Amnioinfusion and the intrauterine prevention of meconium aspiration. Am J Obstet Gynecol 1994; 171:1601–1605.

11. Goodwin TM, Milner-Masterson L, Paul RH. Elimination of fetal scalp blood sampling on a large clinical service. Obstet Gynecol 1994; 83:971–974.

12. Hon EH. An Atlas of Fetal Heart Rate Patterns. Harty Press, New Haven, CT; 1968.

13. Hon EH, Khazin AF. Biochemical studies of the fetus. I. The fetal pH measuring system. Obstet Gynecol 1969; 33:219–236.

14. Johnson JWC, Riley W. Cord blood gas studies: A survey. Clin Obstet Gynecol 1993; 36:99–101.

15. Khazin AF, Hon EH, Hehre FW. Effects of maternal hyperoxia on the fetus. I. Oxygen tension. Am J Obstet Gynecol 1971; 109:628–637.

16. Krebs HB, Petres RE, Dunn LJ, et al. Intrapartum fetal heart rate monitoring. I. Classification and prognosis of fetal heart rate patterns. Am J Obstet Gynecol 1979; 133:762–772.

17. Kubli FW, Hon EH, Khazin AF, Takemura H. Observations on heart rate and pH in the human fetus during labor. Am J Obstet Gynecol 1969; 104:1190–1206.

18. Lauersen NH, Miller FC, Paul RH. Continuous intrapartum monitoring of fetal scalp pH. Am J Obstet Gynecol 1979; 133:44–50.

19. Miyazaki FS, Nevarez F. Saline amnioinfusion for relief of repetitive variable decelerations: A prospective randomized study. Am J Obstet Gynecol 1985; 153:301–306.

20. Parer JT. The current role of intrapartum fetal blood sampling. Clin Obstet Gynecol 1980; 23:565–582.

21. Paul RH, Suidan AK, Yeh SY, Schifrin BS, Hon EH. Clinical fetal monitoring: VII. The evaluation and significance of intrapartum baseline FHR variability. Am J Obstet Gynecol 1975; 123:206–210.

22. Riley RJ, Johnson JWC. Collecting and analyzing cord blood. Clin Obstet Gynecol 1993; 36:13–23.

23. Saling E. Foetal and Neonatal Hypoxia in Relation to Clinical Obstetric Practice. Williams & Wilkins, Baltimore, 1968.

24. Saling E, Schneider D. Biochemical supervision of the foetus during labour. J Obstet Gynaecol Br Commonw 1967; 74:799–811.

25. Smith CV, Nguyen HN, Phelan JP, Paul RH. Intrapartum assessment of fetal well-being: A comparison of fetal acoustic stimulation with acid-base determinations. Am J Obstet Gynecol 1986; 155:726–728.

26. Strong TH, Hetzler G, Sarno AP, Paul RH. Prophylactic intrapartum amnioinfusion: A randomized clinical trial. Am J Obstet Gynecol 1990; 162:1370–1375.

27. Tejani N, Mann LI, Bhakthavathsalan A. Correlation of fetal heart rate patterns and fetal pH with neonatal outcome. Obstet Gynecol 1976; 48:460–463.

28. Wenstrom KD, Parsons MT. The prevention of meconium aspiration in labor using amnioinfusion. Obstet Gynecol 1989; 73:647–651.

29. Westgate J, Garibaldi JM, Greene KR. Umbilical cord blood gas analysis at delivery: a time for quality data. Br J Obstet Gynaecol 1994; 101:1054–1063.

30. Wood C. Fetal scalp sampling: Its place in management. Semin Perinatol 1978; 2:169–179.

31. Wood C, Ferguson R, Leeton J, et al. Fetal heart rate and acid-base status in the assessment of fetal hypoxia. Am J Obstet Gynecol 1967; 98:62–70.

32. Wood C, Newman W, Lumley J, Hammond J. Classification of fetal heart rate in relation to fetal scalp blood measurements and Apgar score. Am J Obstet Gynecol 1969; 105:942–948 .

# Part Four

# INTERPRETATION

# ■ *Chapter Nine*

# Fetal Heart Rate Patterns: Basic and Variant

## I BASIC PATTERNS

The characteristics of the fetal heart rate (FHR) pattern are classified as baseline or periodic/episodic.[17, 18, 33] The baseline features, heart rate and variability, are those recorded between uterine contractions. Periodic changes occur in association with uterine contractions, and episodic changes are those not obviously associated with uterine contractions.

## A Baseline Features

The baseline features of the heart rate are those predominant characteristics which can be recognized between uterine contractions. These consist of the baseline rate and FHR variability.

### BASELINE RATE

The above definition of baseline is adequate in most clinical situations. However, a rigidly described definition suitable for research programs, and computer application is as follows[33]:

Baseline FHR is the approximate mean FHR during a 10-minute segment excluding

1. Periodic or episodic changes.
2. Periods of increased FHR variability.
3. Segments of the baseline which differ by 25 beats/min or more.

In any 10-minute window the minimum baseline duration must be at least 2 minutes, otherwise the baseline for that period is indeterminate. However, baseline can be determined from previous 10-minute segments.

The normal baseline FHR is conventionally considered to be between 110 and 160 beats/min. Values below 110 are termed *bradycardia* and those above 160, *tachycardia*. Baseline bradycardia and tachycardia are quantitated by the actual rate observed, in keeping with the above definition of baseline rate.

## FETAL HEART RATE VARIABILITY

In examining an FHR monitor tracing, in most cases one notes an irregular line. These irregularities demonstrate the FHR variability and represent a slight difference in time interval, and therefore in calculated FHR, from beat to beat (see Chapter 7). If all intervals between heartbeats were identical, the line would be regular or smooth.

Baseline FHR variability is defined as fluctuations in the baseline FHR of 2 cycles/min or greater. These fluctuations are irregular in amplitude and frequency. The sinusoidal pattern differs from variability in that it has a smooth sine wave of regular frequency and amplitude, and is excluded from the definition of FHR variability.

The above definition is adequate for clinical visual interpretation, although in fact two characteristics of FHR variability are recognized. First, short-term variability is considered to be the beat-to-beat fluctuation in heart rate which arises from the fact that there is a slightly different period between R-waves of the electrocardiogram in the normal fetus. The second component is called long-term variability and this can be described as either amplitude excursions or frequency of the longer-term unidirectional changes of FHR which occupy a cycle of less than 1 minute. More rigidly stated definitions of variability suitable for research or computer applications are as follows:

1. Short-term variability is defined as the beat-to-beat changes of fetal heart rate. Thus, for example, if two consecutive beat intervals are slightly different (e.g., 500 ms and 490 ms), they display a small amount of short-term variability. Two consecutive intervals between beats that are substantially different in time length (e.g., 500 ms and 400 ms) have a large amount of short-term variability. If there is no change in the intervals between consecutive beats (e.g., 500 ms and 500 ms), then short-term variability is absent.

2. Long-term variability is defined as the continuous unidirectional change in the baseline FHR over a period of time that encompasses more than adjacent beats. Most authors on this subject do not specify the number of unidirectional changes required to distinguish long-term from short-term variability, but one group arbitrarily decided to accept at least three unidirectional changes and a maximum of 70 unidirectional changes to

the interval, the latter representing 0.5 cycles/min at a heart rate of 140 beats/min.[39] Because under these conditions there must also be a difference in interval length between adjacent beats (even though episodically in one direction), by definition this pattern must also contain short-term variability. Ideally, this should not be the case, since clinically one can observe long-term variability without an associated nonunidirectional short-term variability. Thus, according to these definitions and patterns, short-term variability may exist independently of long-term variability, but long-term variability cannot exist independently of short-term variability. Long-term variability may appear as alterations in the amplitude or the frequency of the complexes.

The most commonly accepted quantitation of long-term variability in North America is the visually determined approximate amplitude range of the fluctuations in long-term variability. Frequency changes in long-term variability have gained little popularity in clinical practice.

# B  Periodic Patterns

Periodic patterns are the alterations in FHR which are associated with uterine contractions. These historically consist of late, early, and variable decelerations, and accelerations. With each of these patterns, the decrease or increase is determined from the most recently determined portion of the baseline.

### LATE DECELERATIONS

Late deceleration of the FHR is a visually apparent gradual decrease (defined as onset of deceleration to nadir of 30 seconds or more) and return to baseline FHR associated with a uterine contraction. It is delayed in timing, with the nadir of the deceleration late in relation to the peak of the contraction.

In most cases the onset, nadir, and recovery are all late in relation to the beginning, peak, and ending of the contraction, respectively.

### EARLY DECELERATIONS

Early deceleration of the FHR is a visually apparent gradual decrease (defined as onset of deceleration to nadir of at least 30 seconds) and return to baseline FHR associated with a uterine contraction. It is coincident in timing, with the nadir of the deceleration coincident to the peak of the contraction.

In most cases the onset, nadir, and recovery are all coincident to the beginning, peak, and ending of the contraction, respectively.

### VARIABLE DECELERATIONS

Variable deceleration is defined as a visually apparent abrupt decrease (defined as onset of deceleration to beginning of nadir of less than 30 seconds) in FHR from the baseline. The decrease in FHR below the baseline is at least 15 beats/min, lasting (from baseline to baseline) at least 15 seconds, and no more than 2 minutes. When variable decelerations are associated with uterine contractions, their onset, depth, and duration commonly vary with successive uterine contractions.

Prolonged deceleration is a subgroup of the variable deceleration, and is defined as an abrupt decrease (defined as onset of deceleration to beginning of nadir of less than 30 seconds) in FHR from the baseline. The decrease in FHR below the baseline is at least 15 beats/min, lasting (from baseline to baseline) at least 15 seconds, and is greater than 2 minutes, but less than 10 minutes. The definition changes to bradycardia if the prolonged deceleration is greater than 10 minutes (see definition of baseline FHR).

## ACCELERATIONS

Acceleration is defined as an abrupt (onset to peak in less than 30 seconds) increase in FHR over baseline of at least 15 beats/min. The duration is at least 15 seconds from the onset to return to baseline, and is no longer than 2 minutes. Before 32 weeks of gestation, accelerations have a peak ≥10 beats/min above the baseline, and last ≥10 seconds.

Prolonged acceleration is of duration greater than 2 minutes and less than 10 minutes. Acceleration of more than 10 minutes represents a baseline change (see definition of baseline FHR).

There is a close association between the presence of accelerations and normal FHR variability.[25] There may be times when it is difficult to decide on whether a pattern is "accelerations," or normal long-term variability complexes. The final decision is not important, as both accelerations and normal variability have the same positive prognostic significance of normal fetal oxygenation.

## QUANTIFICATION CRITERIA OF DECELERATIONS

1. Any deceleration is quantitated by the depth of the nadir in beats per minute below the baseline (excluding transient spikes or electronic artifact). The duration is quantitated in minutes and seconds from the beginning to the end of the deceleration.

2. Decelerations are defined as recurrent if they occur with more than 50 percent of uterine contractions in any 20 minute window.

# C The Normal Pattern

The normal FHR pattern (Fig. 9–1) is accepted as that with a predominant baseline heart rate of between 110 and 160 beats/min. The beat-to-beat variability is present and long-term variability amplitude is between 6 and 25 beats/min. There are no decelerative periodic changes but there may be periodic or episodic accelerations (Fig. 9–2; Table 9–1).

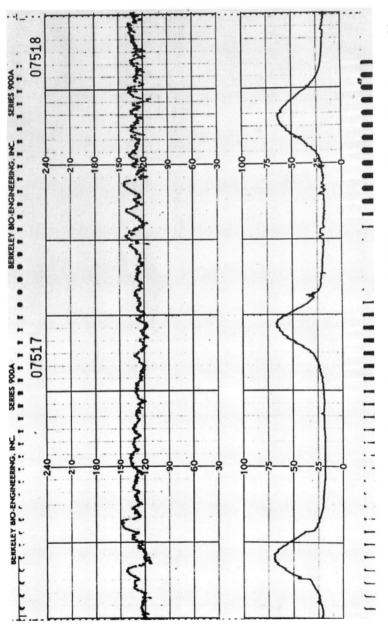

**FIGURE 9–1.** Normal FHR pattern with normal rate (approximately 130 beats/min) and normal short-term and long-term variability (amplitude range approximately 15 beats/min) and absence of periodic changes. This pattern represents a normally oxygenated fetus without evidence of asphyxial stress. Uterine contractions are 2 to 3 minutes apart, with an intensity of approximately 60 mmHg. Vertical sides in the first contraction represent artifact.

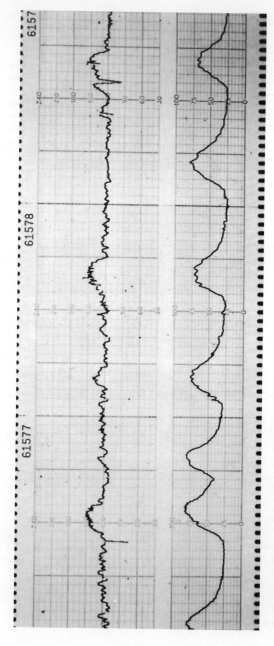

**FIGURE 9–2.** Accelerations with contractions.

**TABLE 9–1.** **Characteristics of Normal Fetal Heart Rate Patterns**

| | |
|---|---|
| Baseline rate | 110 to 160 beats/min |
| Baseline variability (amplitude range) | $\geq 6 \leq 25$ beats/min |
| Periodic patterns | None or accelerations |
| Fetal outcome | Vigorous; Apgar score >7 at 5 minutes |

It is widely accepted in clinical practice that the fetus born with this normal heart rate pattern is virtually always vigorous and normally oxygenated if it is delivered at the time when the normal heart rate pattern is traced.[24, 36, 40, 45] This will, of course, not hold should there be a subsequent traumatic delivery, or should there be a congenital anomaly inconsistent with extrauterine life.

In contrast to this high predictability of fetal normoxia and vigor in the presence of the normal pattern, there are a number of variant patterns which are not so accurately predictive of fetal asphyxia. However, when placed in the context of the clinical case, the progressive change in the patterns, and the duration of the variant patterns, reasonable judgments can be made about the likelihood of fetal asphyxial decompensation. Using this as a screening approach impending intolerable fetal asphyxia can be presumed, or in certain cases, ruled out, by the use of ancillary techniques such as the fetal stimulation test, vibroacoustic stimulation, or fetal blood sampling (see Chapter 8).

---

## II VARIANT FETAL HEART RATE PATTERNS

A number of FHR patterns are seen which, while they are different from the "normal" pattern described above, are certainly not "abnormal." The vast majority of babies born after displaying these patterns have no detectable asphyxial abnormality or sequelae. Therefore these patterns which are not "normal" are termed *variant*.

## A Baseline Rate

### BRADYCARDIA

The initial response of the normal fetus to acute hypoxia or asphyxia is bradycardia.[5] This statement is in contrast to some earlier beliefs where under acutely operated or anesthetized conditions a fetal tachycardia was sometimes noted in response to acutely imposed hypoxia. There is also a report of tachycardia occurring in experimental animals with very mild hypoxia, but clinically and experimentally the initial statement regarding bradycardia holds in the vast majority of cases, because initially the vagal nerve activity is greater than the sympathetic activity.

There are a number of nonasphyxial causes of bradycardia. These include the bradyarrhythmias (e.g., complete heart block), certain drugs (e.g., β-adrenergic blockers or "caine" drugs), or hypothermia. There are other fetuses which have a heart rate below 110 beats/min but are otherwise totally normal and simply represent a normal variation outside our arbitrarily set limits of normal heart rate (Fig. 9–3).

Bradycardia is arbitrarily distinguished from a deceleration which is transient. As defined earlier, a bradycardia is considered to represent a decrease in heart rate below 110 beats/min for 10 minutes or longer.

Prolonged deceleration or bradycardia is considered to represent a prolonged stepwise decrease in fetal oxygenation (Fig. 9–4). This may be a consequence of fetal hypoxia due to vagal activity (and later hypoxic myocardial depression) or the bradycardia may eventually result in fetal hypoxia because of the inability of the fetus to maintain a compensatory increase in stroke volume. As noted above (see Chapter 4) the hypoxic fetus has a certain ability to increase stroke volume in response to bradycardia but this breaks down at severe decreases in heart rate, probably below 60 beats/min. Under these conditions fetal cardiac output cannot be maintained and therefore umbilical blood flow decreases. This results in insufficient oxygen transport from the fetal placenta to the fetal body and therefore may result in eventual fetal hypoxic decompensation.

Reasons for the decreased heart rate may be a stepwise drop in oxygenation such as occurs with maternal apnea or amniotic fluid embolus, a decrease in umbilical blood flow such as occurs with a prolapsed cord, or a decrease in uterine blood flow such as occurs with severe maternal hypotension.

A more complete discussion of specific bradycardias occurs later in this chapter.

## TACHYCARDIA

Tachycardia, an increase or baseline of ≥160 beats/min, is arbitrarily distinguished from an acceleration, or prolonged acceleration, in that its duration is 10 minutes or longer (see definition of baseline FHR).

Tachycardia is seen in some cases in fetal asphyxia but virtually never alone during labor (Fig. 9–5). That is, in the presence of normal FHR variability and absent periodic changes the tachycardia must be assumed to be due to some other cause besides hypoxia. Tachycardia is sometimes seen on recovery from asphyxia and probably represents catecholamine activity following sympathetic nervous or adrenal medullary activity in response to this asphyxial stress, and withdrawal of vagal activity when the hypoxia is relieved.

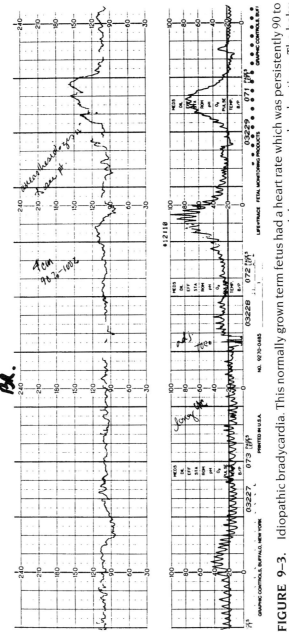

**FIGURE 9–3.** Idiopathic bradycardia. This normally grown term fetus had a heart rate which was persistently 90 to 100 beats/min. FHR variability was normal, accelerations were present, and there were no decelerations. The baby was delivered vaginally and was vigorous at birth.

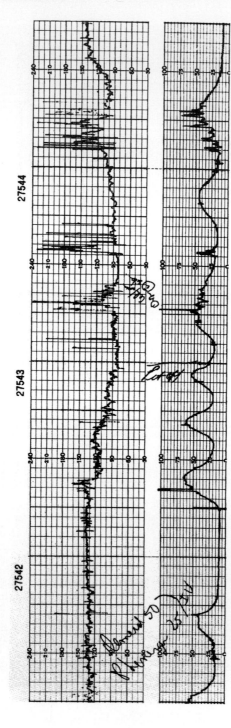

**FIGURE 9–4.** Prolonged fetal bradycardia, probably caused by excessive oxytocin-induced hyperstimulation of the uterus following intravenous meperidine hydrochloride and promethazine hydrochloride into the same tubing. The hyperstimulation and heart rate are returning to normal at the end of the tracing, following appropriate treatment, namely discontinuing oxytocin ("Pit *off*"), maternal administration of oxygen ("O₂6 *L/min*"), and maternal position change ("L *side*"). Note that FHR variability was maintained throughout this asphyxial stress, signifying well-compensated cerebral circulation and oxygenation.

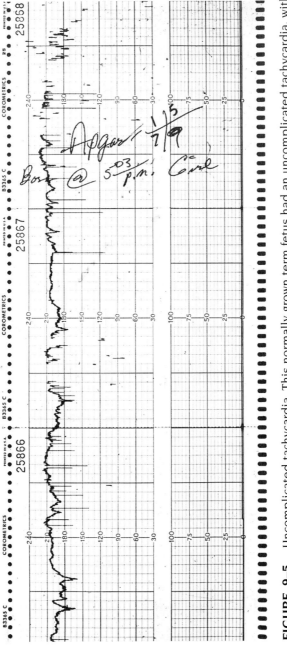

**FIGURE 9–5.** Uncomplicated tachycardia. This normally grown term fetus had an uncomplicated tachycardia, with normal FHR variability and no decelerations. It was vigorous at birth.

There are a number of nonasphyxial causes of tachycardia. The most common of these is maternal or fetal infection, especially chorioamnionitis. Some drugs will cause tachycardia, for example, β-mimetic agents or parasympathetic blockers such as atropine. Tachyarrhythmias occasionally occur and at severe elevations of rate such as above 240 beats/min, these may cause fetal cardiac failure with subsequent hydrops.

## B  Baseline Variability

As noted earlier, in research and mathematical terms, normal FHR variability has two components, short-term and long-term variability. Usually they are both present, and the baseline has a jagged appearance, with unpredictable movements of heart rate up or down. Many clinicians believe that FHR variability is visually determined and quantitated primarily on the basis of long-term rather than short-term complexes, although this is not universally accepted. The absence of either component of FHR variability is considered to be a variant from normal.

There are four basic classes of heart rate variability. They are visually quantitated as the amplitude of the peak-to-trough in beats per minute as follows:

1. Amplitude range undetectable                    absent FHR variability
2. Amplitude range > undetectable
   ≤5 beats/min                                    reduced FHR variability
3. Amplitude range 6 to 25 beats/min               normal FHR variability
4. Amplitude range >25 beats/min                   increased FHR variability

Superimposed on this classification may be the visual estimate of "presence" or "absence" of short-term variability. Generally, both types of variability exist together.

The sinusoidal pattern differs from variability in that it has a smooth sine wave of regular frequency and amplitude, and is excluded from the definition of FHR variability.

The source of FHR variability is clearly complex, with inputs from many cycling physiologic phenomena, including respiratory arrhythmia, blood pressure fluctuations, and thermoregulation, at least in the adult.[21] However, many of the observations are most consistent with the theory that the presence of normal variability requires integrity of the pathways responsible for the production and transmission of variability in (a) the cerebral cortex, (b) the midbrain, (c) the vagus nerve, and (d) the cardiac conduction system[36] (see Fig. 4–9).

It is known that different fetuses have an intrinsic "quantity" of variability, and also that this can change with differences in fetal state[7, 35] (see

Fig. 2–1). It is also known that the components used to describe fetal state can be altered by hypoxia or hypercapnia[3] and by short periods of decreased uterine blood flow.[2, 14] Again, the presence of certain state variables can affect others (e.g., during fetal breathing movements there is a respiratory arrhythmia,[9] and during prelabor myometrial activity there is a change to the quiescent state in fetal sheep).[32] It is important to be aware of such activities in order to make the appropriate distinction between asphyxial and nonasphyxial causes of decreased variability.

As described earlier, in the past FHR variability had been ascribed to an interaction between two branches of the autonomic nervous system— parasympathetic and β-adrenergic—with different time constants. Because variability is primarily transmitted via the parasympathetic nerves in primates, this theory is unlikely to be true.[6, 38] Variability is more likely due to numerous sporadic inputs from various areas of the cerebral cortex and lower centers to the cardiac integratory centers in the medulla oblongata, which are then transmitted down the vagus nerve. Current theory suggests that these inputs decrease in the presence of cerebral asphyxia, so variability decreases after failure of the fetal hemodynamic compensatory mechanisms to maintain cerebral oxygenation.

The most important currently accepted aspect of these clinical correlates is the fact that, in the presence of normal FHR variability, no matter what other FHR patterns may be present, the fetus is not suffering cerebral tissue asphyxia, because it has been able to successfully centralize the available oxygen and is thus physiologically compensated. In the presence of excessive asphyxial stress, however, as evidenced by severe periodic changes or prolonged bradycardia, this compensation may break down, and the fetus may have progressive central tissue asphyxia (i.e., hypoxia in cerebral and myocardial tissues). In this case, it is theorized that FHR variability decreases and eventually is lost.

There are several possible nonasphyxial causes of decreased or absent FHR variability: (a) absence of cortex (anencephaly)[8]; (b) narcotized or drugged higher centers (e.g., by morphine, meperidine, diazepam, magnesium sulfate; Fig. 9–6); (c) vagal blockade (e.g., by atropine or scopolamine; see Fig. 12–3); and (d) defective cardiac conduction system (e.g., complete heart block; see Fig. 7–10).

The essence of the art of appropriate intrapartum FHR interpretation is noting a decrease or disappearance of FHR variability in the presence of appropriate asphyxial stress patterns. Fortunately, the vast majority of fetuses will begin labor with normal FHR variability, so changes can be followed. Also, the ability of the clinician's eye to quantitate FHR variability is excellent when compared to computer programs.[22]

Fetuses with unexplained virtual absence of FHR variability and no periodic changes fall into several categories: (a) quiet sleep state; (b) idio-

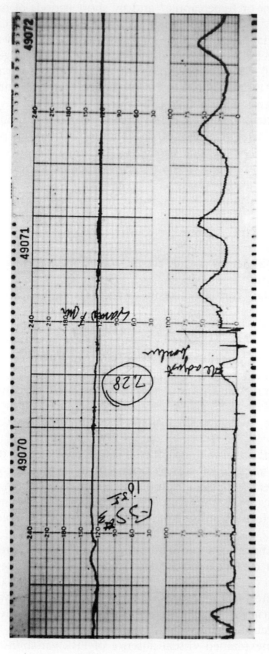

**FIGURE 9–6.** No variability of FHR. The patient was a severe preeclamptic receiving magnesium sulfate and narcotics. The normal scalp blood pH (7.28) assures one that the absence of variability is nonasphyxic in origin and that the fetus is not chronically asphyxiated and decompensating. The uterine activity channel has an inaccurate trace in the first half.

pathic reduced FHR variability, with no obvious explanation, but no evidence of asphyxia or compromised central nervous system (CNS); (c) centrally acting drugs; (d) congenital neurologic abnormality, due to either a developmental CNS defect or acquired from an in utero infection or asphyxial event[20, 34, 41, 46]; or (e) deep asphyxia with inability of the heart to manifest periodic changes. These are further discussed in Chapter 12.

If the FHR variability is reduced, or absent on initial placement of the monitor, this makes the clinician's ability to determine if progressive asphyxia is occurring more difficult, or even impossible, without ancillary testing. Delivery is sometimes expedited to give the fetus the benefit of uncertainty, although there is not consensus that this is the correct approach (see Chapter 12).

# C  Periodic Changes in Fetal Heart Rate

## LATE AND EARLY DECELERATIONS

Late and early decelerations, already defined earlier, have the following characteristics[17, 18] (see Fig. 2–5):

1. They are smooth and rounded in configuration and are the mirror image of the contraction.
2. They are persistent, often occurring with each contraction.
3. Their onset, nadir, and recovery are generally delayed 10 to 30 seconds after the onset, apex, and resolution of the contraction.
4. The depth of the dip is related to the intensity of the contraction.

Late decelerations are of two varieties[15, 27, 30, 36, 37]:

The first type, reflex late deceleration (Fig. 9–7), is sometimes seen when an acute insult (e.g., reduced uterine blood flow due to maternal hypotension) is superimposed on a previously normally oxygenated fetus in the presence of contractions. These late decelerations are caused by a decrease in uterine blood flow (with the uterine contraction), beyond the capacity of the fetus to extract sufficient oxygen. The relatively deoxygenated blood is carried from the fetal placenta through the umbilical vein to the heart and is distributed to the aorta, neck vessels, and head (see Figs. 4–2 to 4–4). Here, the low oxygen tension is sensed by chemoreceptors, and neuronal activity results in a vagal discharge, which causes the transient deceleration (Fig. 9–8). The deceleration is presumed to be "late" because of the circulation time from the fetal placental site to the chemoreceptors and also because the progressively decreasing oxygen tension must reach a certain threshold before vagal activity occurs. There may also be baroreceptor activity causing the vagal discharge.[27] Between contractions, oxygen delivery is adequate and there is no additional vagal activity, so the baseline heart rate is normal.

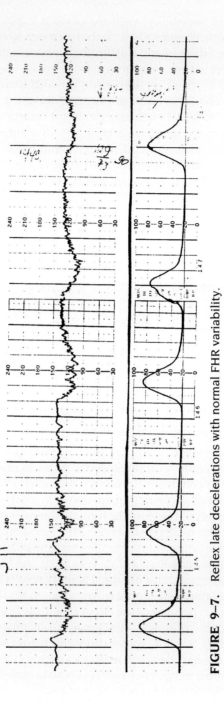

**FIGURE 9–7.** Reflex late decelerations with normal FHR variability.

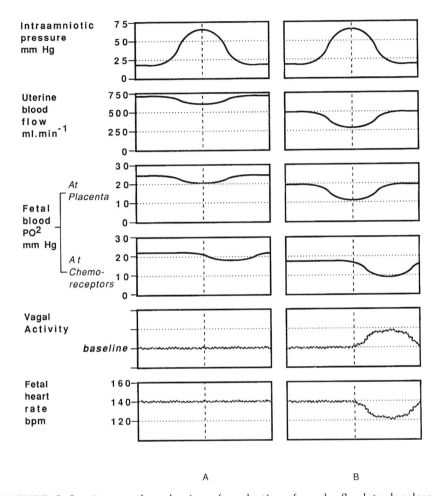

A                    B

**FIGURE 9–8.** Proposed mechanism of production of vagal reflex late decelerations. In most cases there is a small reduction of uterine blood flow (UBF) concomitantly with a uterine contraction. This produces a small reduction in fetal placental blood oxygen tension ($PO_2$), and also, after a period of time for circulation, at the fetal chemoreceptors in the head and neck. A. Under normal conditions the reduction in oxygen tension is insufficient to cause increased vagal activity, so there is no change in FHR. B. However, under conditions of reduced UBF, the fetal oxygen tension is lower, and the reduction with the contraction is greater. This reduction in oxygen tension crosses the threshold for stimulating vagal activity, so we have a rounded reduction and recovery of FHR (i.e., a reflex late deceleration).

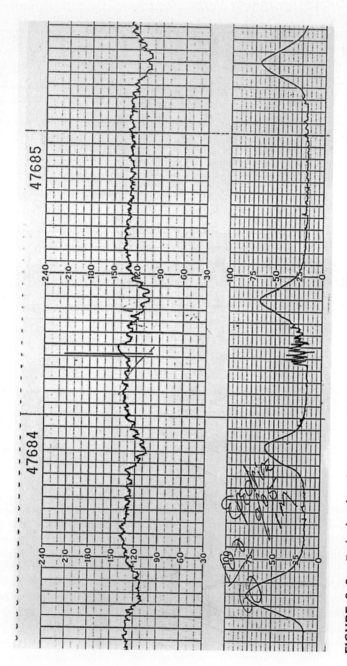

**FIGURE 9–9.**   Early decelerations.

These late decelerations are accompanied by normal FHR variability and thus signify normal CNS integrity (i.e., the fetus is physiologically "compensated" in the vital organs; Fig. 9–7).

The periodic change historically called *early deceleration* appears to simply be a variant of the reflex late deceleration (Fig. 9–9). It is not clear why the deceleration is not late, but early decelerations have been noted to evolve into late decelerations.

The second type of late deceleration is a result of the same initial mechanism, except that the deoxygenated bolus of blood from the placenta is presumed to be insufficient to support myocardial action, so for the period of the contraction there is direct myocardial hypoxic depression (or failure) as well as vagal activity[15, 27] (Fig. 9–10). This variety is seen without variability (Fig. 9–11) signifying fetal "decompensation" (i.e., inadequate fetal cerebral and myocardial oxygenation). It is seen most commonly in states of decreased placental reserve (e.g., with preeclampsia or intrauterine growth retardation or

| | Control | Atropine | Mechanisms |
|---|---|---|---|
| Normoxia | FHR ┌──────┐ UBF ∨ AO | FHR ┌──────┐ UBF AO | Vagal reflex via chemoreceptors |
| Hypoxia | FHR UBF ∨ AO | FHR UBF ∨ AO | Vagal reflex and cardiovascular (myocardial) hypoxic depression |

**FIGURE 9–10.** The proposed mechanism of production of reflex late decelerations (normoxia row) and nonreflex late decelerations (hypoxia row) in fetal sheep. The bar marked AO represents maternal aortic occlusion (reducing uterine blood flow) for 20 seconds. Note that the FHR demonstrates a late deceleration after AO, and that this is abolished by the vagal blocker atropine. There is no change in umbilical blood flow (UBF) or fetal arterial blood pressure, showing that the deceleration is chemoreceptor and not baroreceptor mediated. During maternal hypoxia the late deceleration is deeper and more prolonged, and UBF decreases. Atropine modifies the late deceleration, but does not abolish it, supporting the view that the late deceleration is partially vagal in origin, and also due to reduced circulation, presumably due to hypoxic myocardial depression. (From Harris JL, Krueger TR, Parer JT. Mechanisms of late decelerations of the fetal heart rate during hypoxia. Am J Obstet Gynecol 1982; 144:491–496. Used by permission.)

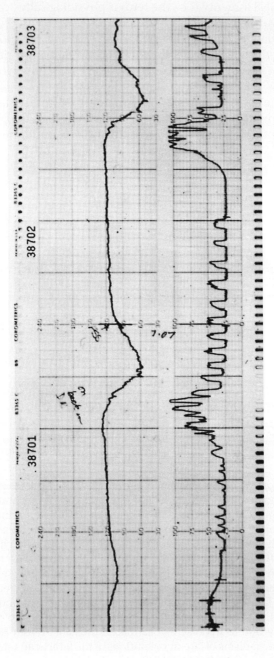

**FIGURE 9–11.**  Late decelerations with virtually absent FHR variability. These findings represent transient asphyxial myocardial failure as well as intermittent vagal decreases in heart rate. The lack of FHR variability also signifies a decreased cerebral oxygenation. Note the acidosis in fetal scalp blood (7.07). A 3340-g girl with Apgar scores of 3 (1 minute) and 4 (5 minutes) was delivered soon after this tracing was made. Cesarean section was considered to be contraindicated because of a severe preeclamptic coagulopathy.

following prolonged asphyxial stresses, such as a long period of severe reflex late decelerations).

The distinguishing feature between reflex and nonreflex late decelerations is therefore the presence of FHR variability in the former. Each category has been shown to dichotomize into two groups based on pH, that of the reflex late deceleration group being in the normal range.[40]

Further support for the two etiologies of late decelerations comes from observations on chronically catheterized fetal monkeys in spontaneous labor during the course of intrauterine death.[30] The animals were initially observed with normal blood gases, normal FHR variability, presence of accelerations and no persistent periodic changes. After a variable period of time they first developed late decelerations, and retained accelerations. This period was associated with a small decline in ascending aortic oxygen tension, from 28 to 24 mmHg, and normal acid-base state. These late decelerations were probably of the vagal reflex type, due to chemoreceptor activity. An average of more than 3 days after the onset of these reflex decelerations, accelerations were lost, in the presence of worsening hypoxia (oxygen tension 19 mmHg) and acidosis (pH 7.22). Fetal death followed an average of 36 hours of persistent late decelerations, and these latter decelerations without accelerations were presumed to be of the nonreflex, myocardial depression type.

Severe late decelerations have been described as those with a drop of more than 45 beats/min below the baseline and may be seen with reflex or nonreflex late decelerations.[26] There are heart rate and duration criteria for identifying mild and moderate late decelerations, but they are mainly of statistical, rather than clinical, importance.

When late decelerations are present, vigorous efforts should be made to eliminate them by optimizing placental blood flows and maternal hyperoxia. Vagal late decelerations, which in most cases are a result of an acute asphyxial episode, can generally be abolished. If not, the fetus may accumulate an oxygen debt, though usually not before 30 minutes in a normally grown fetus who was previously normoxic. However, those late decelerations caused by myocardial failure usually are seen when placental reserve is surpassed and the intermittent decreases in uterine blood flow with each contraction can no longer be tolerated (Fig. 9–12). The abolition of such late decelerations is less likely.

## VARIABLE DECELERATIONS

Variable decelerations (Fig. 9–13), defined earlier, have the following characteristics:

1. The appearance of the dip is variable in duration, depth, and shape from contraction to contraction.

2. Variable decelerations are usually abrupt in onset and cessation, some-

*Text continued on page 170*

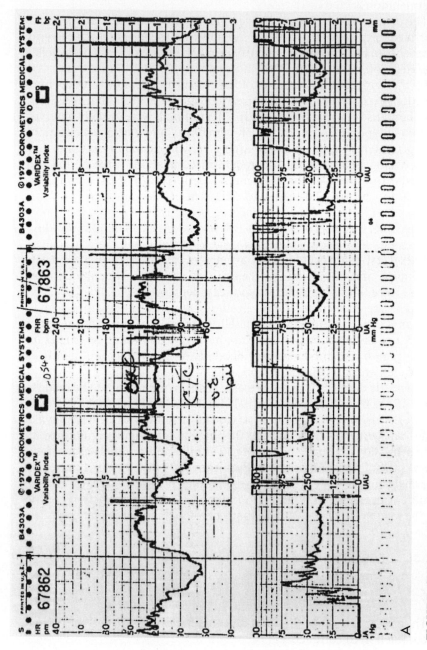

**FIGURE 9–12.** A–C. A case of fetal cardiorespiratory decompensation showing the evolution of the smooth baseline over 30 minutes. In this case the asphyxial stress is manifested as late decelerations. Death occurred in utero about 20 minutes later.

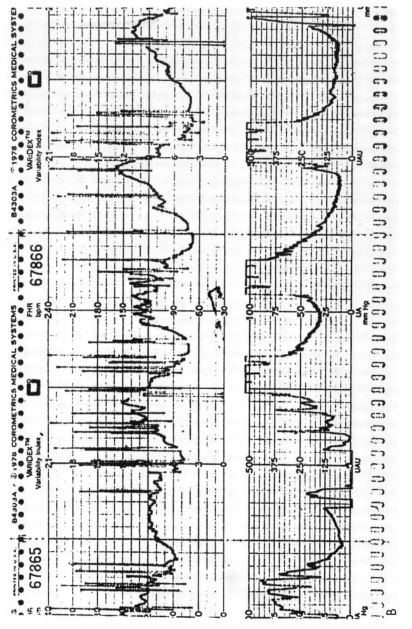

*Illustration continued on following page*

**FIGURE 9–12.** *Continued*

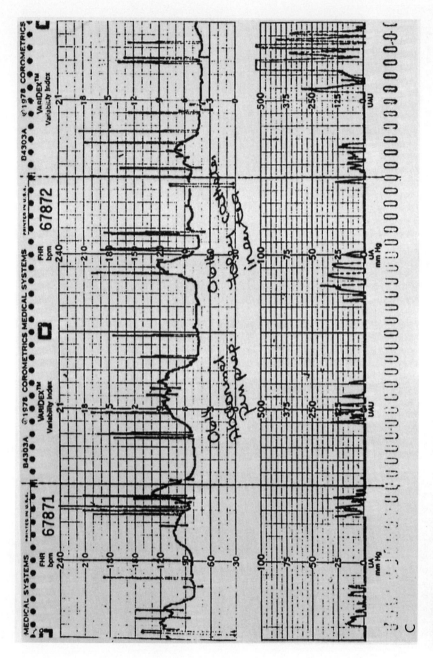

**FIGURE 9–12.** *Continued*

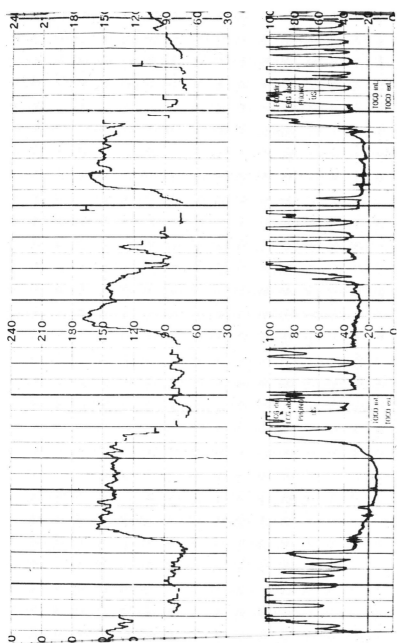

**FIGURE 9–13.** Variable decelerations. Intrapartum recording using fetal scalp electrode and tokodynamometer. The spikes in the uterine activity channel represent maternal pushing efforts in the second stage of labor. Note normal baseline variability between contractions, signifying normal central oxygenation despite the intermittent asphyxial stress represented by the severe variable decelerations.

times falling 60 beats/min in one or several beats. They are thus neurogenic (vagal) in origin.

3. They are described as severe when the decelerations are (a) below 60 beats/min, and (b) longer than 60 seconds in duration. Some authorities have suggested that severity also includes decelerations that are more than 60 beats/min below the baseline heart rate, but this is not so clearly accepted, presumably because it may still be within the ability of the Frank–Starling mechanism to compensate.

4. Variable decelerations without the criteria listed in (3) are classified as mild to moderate.

In addition, other criteria have been proposed, and related to degrees of acidosis.[26]

These abrupt decelerations in heart rate represent the firing of the vagus nerve in response to certain stimuli, either umbilical cord compression, generally in the first stage of labor, or substantial head compression (e.g., during pushing, late in the second stage of labor).[1, 19] Whether the fetus is still normoxic in the central tissues (i.e., physiologically compensated) can be determined by observations of the maintenance of FHR variability.

There are heart rate and duration criteria for mild and moderate variable decelerations, but these classifications are of little importance. The major factor to observe is retention of baseline FHR variability.

The clinical significance of variable decelerations is that they represent a reduction of umbilical blood flow. It is obvious why this is so if they are caused by compression of the umbilical cord. If they are caused by intense vagal activity, then the associated decrease in umbilical blood flow results from a drop in fetal cardiac output because of the relative inability of the fetus to maintain cardiac output at very low heart rates (e.g., below about 60 beats/min; see Chapter 4).

When severe variable decelerations are present, vigorous efforts should be made to abolish them, because it is likely that even the normally grown fetus with normal placental function eventually will decompensate, although usually not before 30 minutes (Fig. 9–14). The normal fetus, however, has a much greater ability to tolerate mild or moderate variable decelerations for a prolonged period.

The theory of variable decelerations being caused by cord compression has given rise to the technique of amnioinfusion[29] (see Chapter 8). In this straightforward technique sterile crystalloid is infused into the amniotic cavity through an intrauterine catheter, with an initial bolus of 250 to 1000 ml and a maintenance of about 2 to 3 ml/mm (see Fig. 8–5). This has been shown to result in a lowered incidence of severe variable decelerations and may allow a vaginal delivery instead of a cesarean section for presumed fetal asphyxia.[48]

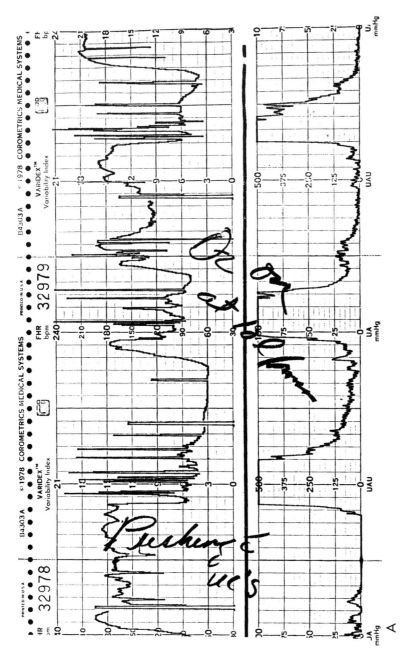

**FIGURE 9–14.** These tracings show a compensated fetus undergoing severe asphyxial stress (i.e., severe variable decelerations) (A), and its eventual decompensation 20 minutes later (B). Delivery was approximately 10 minutes after tracing B. Decompensation is signified by the virtual absence of FHR variability and the smoothness of the decelerations. Apgar scores 0, 0; neonatal death at 4 days of age.

*Illustration continued on following page*

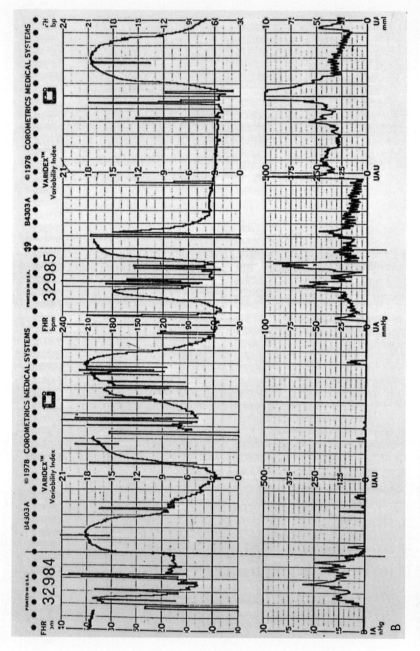

**FIGURE 9–14.** *See legend on page* 171

It may also decrease the incidence of meconium aspiration when the meconium is thick. It appears to be more efficacious in premature fetuses than term fetuses, and is not so effective in the second stage of labor, lending support to the theory that second-stage variable decelerations are due to head and not cord compression.

## ACCELERATIONS WITH CONTRACTIONS

Accelerations sometimes occur with uterine contractions (see Fig. 9–2) and have no adverse prognostic significance. They are probably similar to the accelerations that are seen with fetal movement in the antepartum period, and thus are indicative of a reactive and healthy fetus. Accelerations with contractions probably represent the net result of greater sympathetic activity than parasympathetic activity during contractions in the case of a particular fetus.

"Shoulders" and the "overshoot" pattern probably represent a combination of sympathetic and vagal activity, with the sympathetic being predominant when the shoulders or overshoot occurs. There is no sound evidence that they have any prognostic significance, and if they are seen in the absence of FHR variability, their presence is subservient to this observation.

---

# III THE INFLUENCE OF IN UTERO TREATMENT

It is now well recognized that fetal oxygenation can be improved, acidosis relieved, and variant FHR patterns abolished by certain modes of treatment. The events that result in fetal stress (recognized by FHR patterns) are presented in Table 8–2, together with the recommended treatment maneuvers and presumed mechanisms for improving fetal oxygenation. These should be the primary maneuvers carried out, and if the hypoxic insult is acute and the fetus was previously normoxic, there is an excellent chance that the variant FHR pattern will be abolished. Late decelerations, if present, are most likely of the reflex type, rather than caused by myocardial failure.

During labor an FHR pattern with decreasing variability due to asphyxia is virtually always preceded by a heart rate pattern signifying asphyxial stress [e.g., late decelerations, variable decelerations (usually severe), or a prolonged bradycardia]. In the antepartum period, however, before the onset of uterine contractions, this does not necessarily hold, and a fetus may develop decreasing or absent variability without periodic or baseline FHR changes. In addition, the normal evolution to decreased or absent variability sometimes occurs with relatively minor decelerations in cases of chorioamnionitis, and dysmaturity.

If the FHR patterns cannot be improved (i.e., if the stress patterns indicative of peripheral tissue or central tissue asphyxia persist for a significant period), further diagnosis or delivery may be indicated.

Certain patterns are of such a severe character that immediate delivery without ancillary testing, such as fetal scalp sampling, is warranted if they cannot rapidly be relieved. They include patterns with a smooth baseline and severe, uncorrectable late or variable decelerations (Figs. 9–15 and 9–16), or a prolonged bradycardia below 60 beats/min with a smooth baseline (see Fig. 11–3). Such fetuses may be presumed to be either already asphyxiated or soon to become so.

---

# IV OTHER PATTERNS

A number of patterns do not fit simply into the category of "basic patterns." They are less common, and their significance is generally more controversial.

## A Bradycardias

As noted previously, bradycardia is defined as a baseline heart rate below 110 beats/min for 10 minutes. This is to distinguish it from *deceleration,* which refers to a decrease in FHR below 110 beats/min for less than 10 minutes. These criteria are, of course, arbitrary and have been developed primarily for communication rather than based strictly on a physiologic foundation.

It has already been pointed out that there are a number of clearly nonasphyxial causes of a persistent FHR below 110 beats/min (e.g., see Figs. 7–10 and 9–3).

A number of labels have been placed on various bradycardias, reflecting their appearance, occurrence, or presumed etiology (e.g., prolonged brady-cardia, prolonged end-stage bradycardia, and post-paracervical block brady-cardia).

### PROLONGED BRADYCARDIA OR PROLONGED DECELERATION

Moderate bradycardia (i.e., not below 100 beats/min) may represent continuous head compression and therefore vagal activity. The reason for the vagal response to head compression is uncertain, but it may be caused by cerebral ischemia.[17] It may also be caused by stimulation of the dura. Provided that FHR variability is maintained, prolonged moderate bradycardia is not associated with fetal depression. Some fetuses with moderate bradycardia may simply have rates below the arbitrary level of 110 beats/min.

Prolonged deceleration or bradycardia is generally applied to a sudden drop from a normal FHR to values below 110 beats/min, especially below 80 beats/min. As mentioned previously, bradycardia is the initial response of the

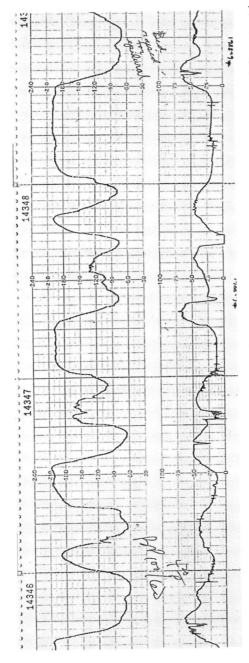

**FIGURE 9–15.** A sinister heart rate pattern in a 28-week fetus (gestational age determined after delivery) with baseline tachycardia, absence of heart rate variability, and severe periodic changes. The scalp blood pH was 7.0, and the fetus died shortly after this tracing. Cesarean section was not performed because the fetus was believed to be previable, although in fact it was 1100 g. There is much artifact in the uterine activity channel.

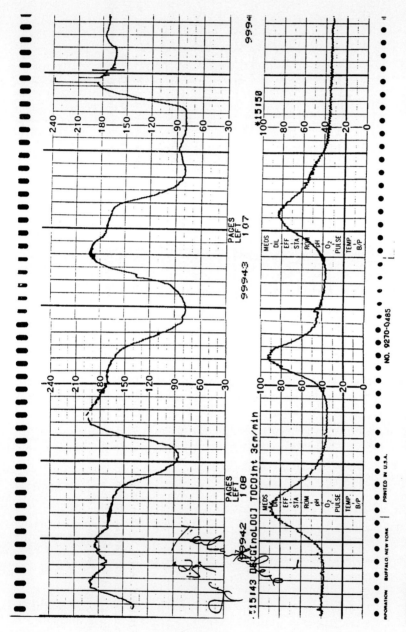

**FIGURE 9–16.**   This FHR pattern of profound decelerations and absent FHR variability must be considered to represent serious asphyxia unless it can be ruled out by ancillary testing, such as fetal scalp sampling. The presence of overshoot does not alter this presumed diagnosis. Because the majority of such fetuses are, in fact, deeply asphyxiated, emergent delivery is recommended.

fetus to acute asphyxia. It is probably a vagal response to peripheral or central chemoreceptor activity. The asphyxic stimulus may be caused by (1) a decrease in maternal oxygen tension, such as during the apnea of a seizure; (2) a decrease in uterine blood flow, such as during excessive uterine contractions or acute maternal hypotension; (3) a decrease in umbilical blood flow, such as by cord compression (Fig. 9–17); or (4) loss of placental area, such as in abruptio placentae. The extent of the bradycardia depends on the degree of fetal hypoxia. There may also be a baroreceptor influence causing the bradycardia with prolongation of asphyxia.

In rare cases, a prolonged bradycardia is the result of fetal hemorrhage, usually catastrophic, such as tearing of vasa previa or rupture of an anomalous fetal placental vessel. In such cases the fetus may be born not only asphyxiated but in hemorrhagic shock.

Immediately upon recognition of a bradycardia, attempts should be made to optimize fetal oxygenation by maintenance of maternal blood pressure, avoidance of excessive uterine activity, position change, hydration, and possibly, maternal hyperoxia (see Table 8–2). There is no need for grave concern if moderate bradycardia is not abolished. However, if the heart rate is below 100 beats/min, more vigorous efforts should be made to alleviate it, even in the presence of good FHR variability. An acute drop in heart rate to less than 60 beats/min usually results in fetal asphyxial decompensation, and it becomes an obstetric emergency to abolish it or deliver the baby before severe central asphyxia occurs (Fig. 9–18).

Fortunately, most sudden bradycardias resolve spontaneously or with various positional changes. However, they are of sufficient concern that many women whose babies exhibit several prolonged bradycardic episodes are brought to the delivery room for labor, in case the FHR does not recover after one of them. On rare occasions the bradycardia does not resolve, and the infants may be deeply depressed owing to asphyxia (Fig. 9–19). Such cases are seen more commonly in postdate pregnancies and, fortunately, are rare. The etiology of the bradycardia is not always apparent, and some have ascribed it to excessive vagal activity.

### PROLONGED END-STAGE BRADYCARDIA

This term refers to a prolonged deceleration, generally late in the second stage of labor, in the presence of an otherwise normal FHR tracing (Fig. 9–20).[16] This pattern is not uncommon, and will be seen much more frequently if one adopts the practice of monitoring in the delivery room and continuing to monitor FHR until the time of delivery.

Prolonged end-stage bradycardia is quite likely to be a vagal response to head compression as the head traverses the depths of the pelvis. Compression may cause a decrease in cerebral blood flow and brief local ischemia, which could produce a vagal response. Alternatively, the vagal discharge may be caused by compression of the dura. *Text continued on page 182*

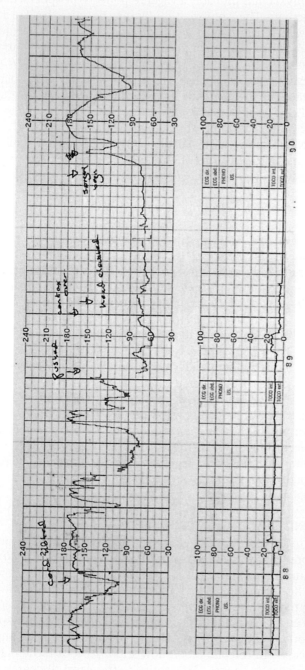

**FIGURE 9–17.** Prolonged deceleration resulting from prolapsed cord ("*cord noted*") in a premature baby at 29 weeks of gestation. Delivery was attempted during a single push with contraction, and, when this effort failed, cesarean section was performed. The 1460-g girl had Apgar scores of 5 (1 minute) and 5 (5 minutes) and did well.

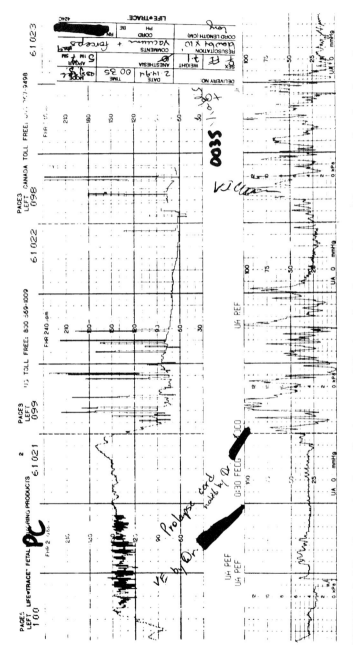

**FIGURE 9–18.** Severe bradycardia due to umbilical cord prolapse. The rapid response by the obstetric team included application of the vacuum extractor and forceps, and a decision–delivery time of about 4 minutes. The 3180-g newborn girl had Apgar scores of 5 (1 minute) and 7 (5 minutes).

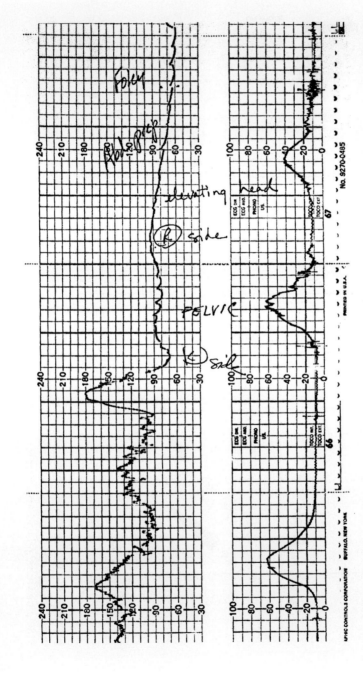

**FIGURE 9–19.** A sudden prolonged unremitting bradycardia, with lack of variability in a postdate (42 weeks) patient. The fetus was delivered by emergency cesarean section 9 minutes after the start of the deceleration, with Apgar scores of 2 (1 minute) and 3 (5 minutes).

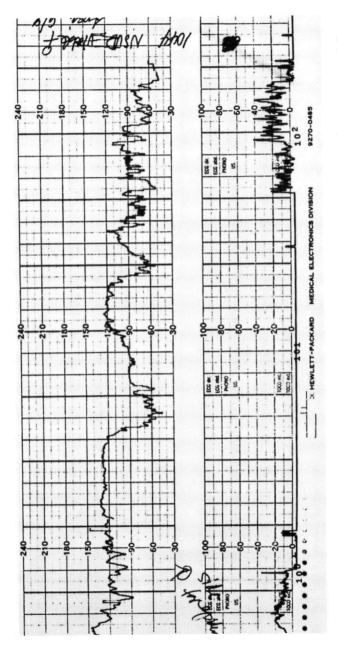

**FIGURE 9–20.** A prolonged end-stage bradycardia, with retention of FHR variability, and spontaneous delivery of a vigorous fetus, Apgar scores 6 (1 minute) and 9 (5 minutes).

These patterns were in the past generally managed by rapid termination of labor, either by forceps or encouragement to push. As with the spontaneous prolonged bradycardias, however, the results of expectant management have not been well tested. Position change (which is somewhat limited in the second stage) and discouragement from pushing sometimes appear to result in resolution of prolonged bradycardia. Elevation of the fetal head may also be efficacious, but studies purporting to demonstrate the benefit of the maneuver suffer from the defect of having no equivalent untreated group.

The current recommendation is that if the bradycardia is persistent and FHR variability decreases, the baby should be delivered as rapidly as possible. However, if variability is retained, efforts should be made to abolish the bradycardia or effect a spontaneous delivery. It is unusual for this pattern to result in absence of FHR variability and fetal decompensation in less than 10 minutes, if the FHR is above 60 beats/min.

## POST-PARACERVICAL BLOCK BRADYCARDIA

Paracervical block for labor has decreased concomitantly with the increased availability of epidural anesthesia for relief in labor. However, it is still used, and the earlier experience with it will be reviewed.

On the average, bradycardia occurs 7 minutes after paracervical block is administered and lasts 8 minutes (Fig. 9–21). The range in both of these values, the degree of bradycardia, and the associated FHR changes are quite variable. Its incidence varies from 0 to 56 percent, depending on drug, dosage, and definition. An average incidence is 15 percent. Some fetal deaths have been associated with paracervical block bradycardia.[43]

Although the etiology is controversial, the most likely cause of the bradycardia is a direct fetal toxic reaction to the local anesthetic drug, not necessarily because of direct fetal injection but because of rapid uptake of the drug by the fetus, possibly via the uterine arteries. Fetal levels of such a drug can be quite high, though rarely higher than that of the mother. A further theory is that the local anesthetic agent causes spasm of the uterine arteries, resulting in decreased uterine blood flow and, hence, fetal hypoxia. Acidosis has been demonstrated by blood sampling in affected fetuses during the bradycardia.[43]

Minimization of this undesirable side effect of paracervical block is assisted by using minimal quantities of drugs. Careful technique to ensure that the drug is placed just submucosally will avoid inadvertent fetal injection. Paracervical block is considered to be contraindicated if the fetus already has a fetal heart rate pattern suggestive of asphyxia.

If bradycardia does develop, supportive management is recommended (i.e., position change and maternal hyperoxia) until it resolves. If the pattern does resolve and FHR returns to normal, no further evaluation is needed, but subsequent paracervical injection should be avoided.

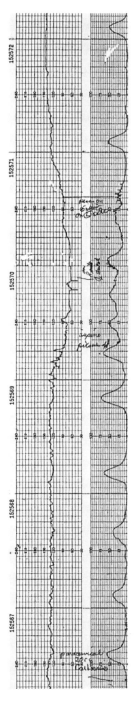

**FIGURE 9–21.** A prolonged deceleration following paracervical block anesthesia with 20 ml of carbocaine. Note the onset approximately 10 minutes after administration and the resolution after approximately 8 minutes. The deceleration is coincident with uterine hypertonus and tachysystole. (From Paul RH. Intrapartum monitoring case examples. Los Angeles County-University of Southern California Medical Center, 1971. Used by permission.)

Except in rare and profoundly abnormal cases, delivery should be avoided during the bradycardia, because the fetus is better able to get rid of the drug transplacentally than to detoxify it postnatally.

# B  Arrhythmias

Numerous fetal arrhythmias have been diagnosed in utero.[47] These include complete heart block, premature atrial contractions, premature ventricular contractions, bigeminy, supraventricular tachycardia, paroxysmal atrial tachycardia, blocked atrial premature beats, atrial flutter, and asystole of variable duration.

The FHR monitor detects and depicts the interval between beats and is thus a very sensitive dysrhythmia detector. Bradyarrhythmias are the most commonly reported. Complete heart block appears as an FHR of approximately 50 to 60 beats/min, with virtually absent FHR variability (see Fig. 7–10).

Bradycardias and tachycardias may be doubled or halved by the cardiotachometer, particularly in the Doppler mode. This artifact can almost always be ruled out by brief auscultation (see Chapter 7).

Arrhythmias generally represent cardiac conduction defects which have an anatomic or functional basis. The persistent types appear to have a worse prognosis than the intermittent ones, the latter often resolving in the newborn.

Complete heart block has an incidence of about 1 in 20,000 births, and approximately 30 percent of cases are associated with heart disease, often a cardiac structural abnormality. About 10 percent of newborns with congenital heart block die in early infancy.

An infant with heart block may have a mother with collagen vascular disease, particularly systemic lupus erythematosis, so such women should be screened appropriately.

The extreme tachycardias, generally above 240 beats/min, have sometimes been associated with hydrops, apparently because of intrauterine cardiac failure. There are case reports of in utero treatments with digoxin, β-adrenergic blocking agents, procainamide, or calcium channel blockers. In some cases there has been resolution of the hydrops.

A great deal of concern was experienced in the past over the fetus with an arrhythmia. It has become obvious that only rarely are early interventions required and most of these infants can tolerate labor well. The most common arrhythmia, intermittent premature beats, need no particular workup besides a routine sonogram. Echocardiography may be helpful in diagnosing the condition and determining whether there are any obvious structural abnormalities before birth in persistent arrhythmia.

The major problem in the fetus with a persistent severe arrhythmia is generally in the newborn period. Such infants should be delivered in a tertiary care center with immediate access to pediatric cardiology care. Those with heart block may need cardiac pacing and those with a tachycardia may need digitalizing to prevent cardiac failure.

# C Sinusoidal Pattern

This is a regular, smooth sine wave-like baseline, with a frequency of approximately 3 to 6/min and an amplitude range of up to 30 beats/min. The regularity of the waves distinguishes it from long-term variability complexes, which are crudely shaped and irregular. Another distinguishing feature is the absence of beat-to-beat or short-term variability (Figs. 9–22 and 9–23).

The pattern was first described in a group of severely affected Rh-isoimmunized fetuses[44] but has subsequently been noted in association with fetuses that are anemic for other reasons, and in asphyxiated infants. It has also been described in cases of normal infants born without depression or acid-base abnormalities, although in these cases there is dispute about whether the patterns are truly sinusoidal or whether, because of the moderately irregular pattern, they are variants of long-term variability. Such patterns, often called *pseudosinusoidal,* are also sometimes seen after administration of narcotics to the mother (Fig. 9–24). It is believed that an essential characteristic of the sinusoidal pattern is extreme regularity and smoothness.

Murata et al.[31] have implicated arginine vasopressin in the sinusoidal pattern. Sinusoidal FHR patterns and increased argine vasopressin blood levels were produced in fetal lambs by hemorrhage, and by arginine vasopressin infusion into vagotomized or atropinized fetuses. These authors proposed that the direct effect of arginine vasopressin on the sinus node may have affected calcium transfer, resulting in the pattern.

The presence of a sinusoidal pattern or variant of this in an Rh-sensitized patient usually suggests anemia with a fetal hematocrit of lower than 30 percent.[28, 42] The presence of hydrops in such a fetus suggests a fetal hematocrit of 15 percent or less. Many severely anemic Rh-affected fetuses do not have a sinusoidal pattern, but rather a rounded, "blunted" pattern, and accelerations are usually absent.

If a sinusoidal pattern is seen in an Rh-sensitized patient and severe hemolysis is confirmed (e.g., by cordocentesis or the Delta OD 450 determination in amniotic fluid), rapid intervention is needed. It may take the form of delivery or possibly intrauterine transfusion, depending on the gestational age and the preceding Rh data, treatment, and work-up.

Management in the absence of Rh disease is somewhat more difficult to recommend. If the pattern is persistent, monotonously regular, and unaccompanied by short-term variability and it cannot be abolished by the maneuvers just described, further workup and evaluation of adequacy of fetal oxygenation (e.g., contraction stress test, fetal stimulation test, biophysical

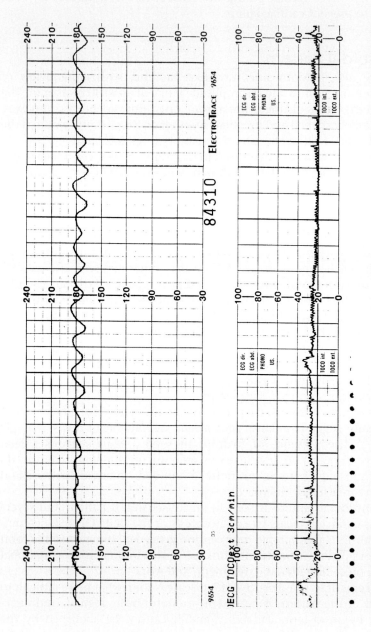

**FIGURE 9–22.** Sinusoidal heart rate pattern in a case of presumed fetal-maternal bleeding at 39 weeks of gestation. Fetal movement was absent, and the fetus was anemic, hematocrit 20 percent. Umbilical arterial pH at birth was 7.19, and base excess −8 mEq • L$^{-1}$ .

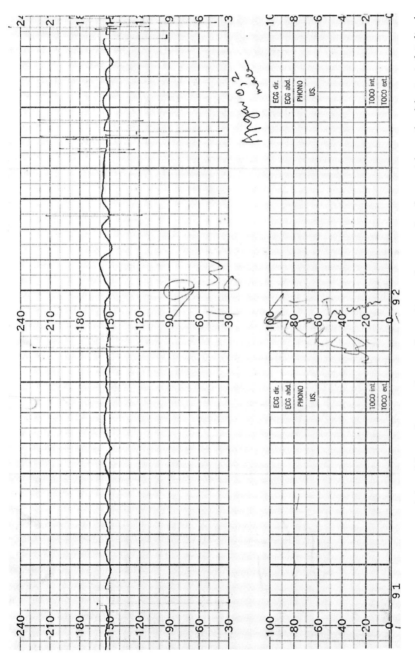

**FIGURE 9–23.** Sinusoidal or "blunted" FHR obtained on a 37-weeks gestation fetus with erythroblastosis fetalis due to Rh isoimmunization, with anemia, hematocrit 21 percent, and acidosis, pH 7.03. The fetus was delivered by cesarean section and has developed normally.

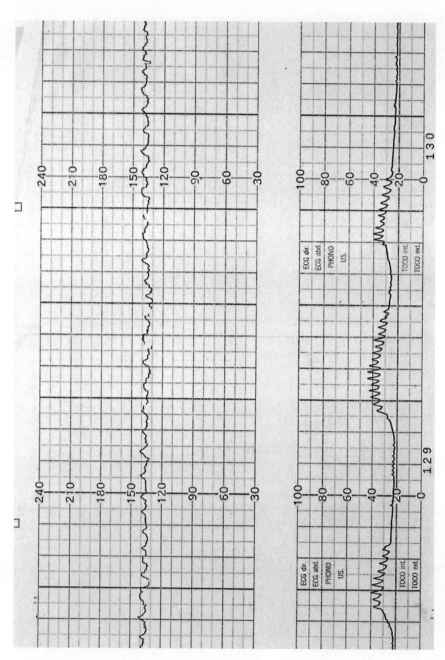

**FIGURE 9–24.** Pseudosinusoidal pattern following maternal administration of alphaprodine (Nisentil). The irregularity of the sine waves distinguishes this pattern from a true sinusoidal pattern.

profile, or fetal blood sampling) is indicated. Nonalloimmune sinusoidal patterns have been associated with severe fetal asphyxia and fetal anemia due to fetal–maternal bleeding, the latter of which can be supported by fetal red cells in maternal blood, detected by the Kleihauer–Betke test.

The presence of sinusoidal patterns in cases of fetal–maternal bleeding, and the less striking blunted variant in Rh-affected babies, has given rise to the view that acute anemia, rather than a slow development of anemia as seen usually with erythoblastosis fetalis, is necessary for the production of the true sinusoidal pattern. As yet there is little evidence for this theory. However, it is consistent with the hormonal causation of the pattern.

If the pattern is irregularly sinusoidal or "pseudosinusoidal," intermittently present, and not associated with intervening periodic decelerations, it is very unlikely to indicate fetal compromise. Hence, immediate delivery is not warranted. The aforementioned ancillary tests may assist in confirming normality in such cases.

## D  Saltatory Pattern

This pattern consists of rapid variations in FHR with a frequency of 3 to 6/min and an amplitude range greater than 25 beats/min (Fig. 9–25). It is qualitatively described as excessive variability, and the variations have a strikingly bizarre appearance.

The saltatory pattern was associated with low Apgar scores in early observations of FHR variability, but it was not possible to relate the time course of the pattern to the fetal depression.[13] This is, fetuses with the pattern in the intrapartum period had a tendency toward low Apgar scores, but it was not clear whether the pattern was present immediately before delivery, or whether it preceded an evolution to a more serious FHR pattern.

The saltatory pattern is almost invariably seen during labor rather than in the antepartum period.

The etiology is uncertain. Clinical experience suggests, however, that it may be similar to that of the increased FHR variability seen in animal experiments with brief and acute hypoxia in the previously normoxic fetus. This increase is presumed to result from an increase in α-adrenergic activity, of which the primary function is to cause selective vasoconstriction of certain vascular beds. A secondary effect of this increased α-adrenergic activity may be excessive variability.

Because it is believed that the fetus with this pattern is hemodynamically compensated, (although it may be mildly hypoxemic) we recommend that attempts be made to abolish it, by maneuvers such as lateral positioning, avoidance of hypotension, avoidance of excessive uterine activity, and perhaps maternal hyperoxia. The pattern is probably similar in significance to mild or moderate variable decelerations.

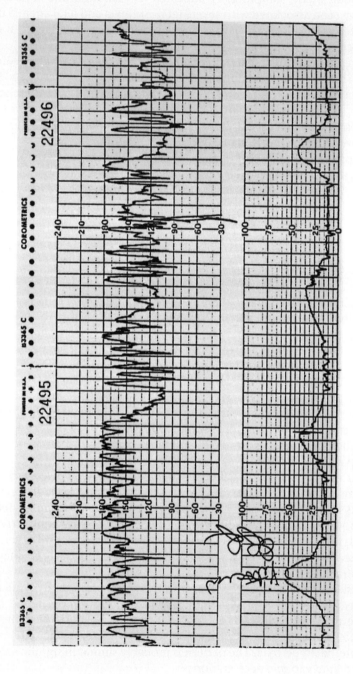

**FIGURE 9-25.** Saltatory pattern showing excessive FHR variability of up to 60 beats/min in brief intervals, probably representing mild hypoxic stress.

# E  The Premature Fetus

Several investigators have examined both the antepartum and intrapartum FHR patterns of the premature and their relationship to fetal blood acid-base status.[4, 49] There now seems little doubt that the same general criteria used in the term fetus can be used for the premature. It has been stated in the past that prematures can quickly develop abnormal patterns and that these patterns tend to progress in severity much more rapidly than in the term fetus. However, we are still awaiting proof of this assertion.

There are some commonly held and erroneous beliefs with regard to prematures. The first is that prematures normally have tachycardia. In fact, the average heart rate of the 28-week-old fetus is about 150 beats/min, with a range of about 130 to 170 beats/min (i.e., only slightly above that of the term fetus). The second is that premature heart rates have "flat baselines." Most prematures have normal FHR variability, and its disappearance or absence should be managed as for a term fetus. There is, however, a tendency for prematures to have a smaller amplitude of variability, and a lower amplitude of accelerations.[11] There is also a widely held belief that prematures tend to have more episodic small variable decelerations.

The response of the premature fetus to vibroacoustic stimulation is also different from that of the term fetus.[10] The percentage of reactive nonstress tests following vibroacoustic stimulation is 90 percent or more above 26 weeks, but only 20 percent or less below this gestational age.

# F  Congenital Anomalies

Except as described for the arrhythmias, the majority of fetuses with congenital anomalies have normal FHR patterns and a response to asphyxia similar to that of the normal fetus. There are several exceptions (e.g., complete heart block and anencephaly). Thus, aneuploid fetuses, such as those with Down's syndrome and trisomy 18, and fetuses with aplastic lungs, meningomyelocele, and hydrocephalus, may give no FHR warning of defects. In one series it was noted that although there was no pathognomonic pattern in such fetuses, the rate of cesarean section for fetal distress was significantly increased.[12]

An important exception is seen with Potter's syndrome. Affected fetuses are generally recognized as growth-retarded because of the oligohydramnios and in addition may have substantial variable decelerations, presumably for the same reason; that is, umbilical cord compression is more likely without the "padding" of adequate amniotic fluid. A number of such fetuses have been delivered by cesarean section for "fetal distress," with the tragic outcome being rapid neonatal death due to hypoplastic lungs.

There is no simple solution to the problem of heroic intervention (generally cesarean section) for the fetus who is destined to be severely defective or to die in the neonatal period. Genetic evaluation and high-resolution ultrasound in certain high-risk groups may decrease the incidence of such problems, but in the case of a youthful primipara without significant family history of genetic disease, screening is not yet available, except possibly for open neural tube defects via α-fetoprotein measurements, and for some aneuploidy within the expanded maternal serum screen.

Even the advances in ultrasonography for visualizing the fetus may be of borderline help during labor, because imaging may not indicate that a fetus has a lethal defect at this stage. Such defects as severe hydrocephalus and renal agenesis would fit this category, but many other defective fetuses, especially those with metabolic disorders or tracheal and other soft tissue abnormalities, often are not identified.

## G  "Shoulders" and "Overshoot"

These terms are used to describe transient increases in FHR either preceding or immediately following a deceleration. They have an undeserved bad reputation. They simply represent the transient net result of dominance of sympathetic over parasympathetic activity. Others believe the shoulders may result from mild cord compression during which only the umbilical vein is compressed; this would produce a temporary fetal hypovolemia. The author believes that the shoulders do not represent an asphyxial stress, and that any fetal compromise results from the associated decelerations. As with all patterns, the significance of the presence or absence of shoulders is secondary to the retention of FHR variability. In the example in Figure 9–16, the shoulders neither ameliorate nor add to the diagnosis of presumed severe fetal asphyxia.

## H  Infection

The presence of infection, particularly chorioamnionitis, is often associated with a tachycardia. This is usually an uncomplicated tachycardia, meaning that the baseline FHR is above 160 beats/min, but the variability is normal, accelerations usually present, and periodic changes absent. However, there is a tendency for variability to be concomitantly reduced with tachycardia.

Anecdotal evidence suggests another disturbing aspect of some cases of fetal infection, and that is an atypical evolution of FHR patterns. That is, the FHR pattern may evolve from a tachycardia with somewhat reduced FHR variability to one with mild late decelerations with reduced variability, and finally a profound bradycardia without variability. As noted above and in Chapter 11, this expected evolution would normally follow deep late or variable decelerations, or a bradycardia.

*Listeria* amnionitis has also been seen with patterns normally associated with fetal asphyxia (i.e., late decelerations without FHR variability).[23] It has been theorized that these patterns were produced not by global asphyxia, but rather cardiogenic and septic shock due to overwhelming fetal sepsis. This same mechanism may well apply to non-*Listeria* infection findings noted above.

Babies with these patterns are usually depressed (i.e., low Apgar scores) but may only have moderate acidosis. Nevertheless, our current opinion is that these babies will benefit from early delivery, so that extrauterine support can be instituted. The major management difficulty with these cases is timely recognition of the severity of the fetal condition despite the atypical evolution of the FHR pattern.

## REFERENCES

1. Ball RH, Parer JT. The physiological mechanisms of variable decelerations. Am J Obstet Gynecol 1992; 166:1683–1689.

2. Bocking AD, Harding R. Effects of reduced uterine blood flow on electrocortical activity, breathing, and skeletal muscle activity in fetal sheep. Am J Obstet Gynecol 1986; 154:655–662.

3. Boddy K, Dawes GS, Fisher R, et al. Foetal respiratory movements, electrocortical and cardiovascular responses to hypoxaemia and hypercapnia in sheep. J Physiol (Lond) 1974; 243:599–618.

4. Bowes WA, Gabbe SG, Bowes C. Fetal heart rate monitoring in premature infants weighing 1500 grams or less. Am J Obstet Gynecol 1980; 137:791–796.

5. Court DJ, Parer JT. Experimental studies of fetal asphyxia and fetal heart rate interpretation. In Nathanielsz PW, Parer JT, eds. Research in Perinatal Medicine (I). Perinatology Press, New York, 1984, pp. 113–169.

6. Dalton KJ, Dawes GS, Patrick JE. The autonomic nervous system and fetal heart rate variability. Am J Obstet Gynecol 1983; 146:456–462.

7. Dawes GS, Fox HE, Leduc BM, et al. Respiratory movements and rapid eye movement sleep in the foetal lamb. J Physiol 1972; 220:119–143.

8. DeHaan J, van Bemmel JH, Stolte LAM, et al. Quantitative evaluation of fetal heart rate patterns II. The significance of fixed heart rate pattern during pregnancy and labor. Eur J Obstet Gynec 1971; 3:103–113.

9. Divon MY, Yeh S-Y, Zimmer EZ, et al. Respiratory sinus arrhythmia in the human fetus. Am J Obstet Gynecol 1985; 151:425–428.

10. Druzin ML, Edershein TG, Hutson JM, Bond AL. The effect of vibroacoustic stimulation on the nonstress test at gestational ages of thirty-two weeks or less. Am J Obstet Gynecol 1989; 161:1476–1478.

11. Druzin ML, Fox A, Kogut E, Carlson C. The relationship of the nonstress test to gestational age. Am J Obstet Gynecol 1985; 153:386–389.

12. Garite TJ, Linzey EM, Freeman RK, Dorchester W. Fetal heart rate patterns and fetal distress in fetuses with congenital anomalies. Obstet Gynecol 1979; 53:716–720.

13. Hammacher K, Huter KA, Bokelmann J, Werners PH. Foetal heart frequency and perinatal condition of foetus and newborn. Gynaecologia (Basel) 1968; 166:348–360.

14. Harding R, Poore ER, Cohen GL. The effect of brief episodes of diminished uterine blood flow on breathing movements, sleep states and heart rate in fetal sheep. J Dev Physiol 1982; 3:231–243.

15. Harris JL, Krueger TR, Parer JT. Mechanisms of late decelerations of the fetal heart rate during hypoxia. Am J Obstet Gynecol 1982; 144:491–496.

**16.** Herbert CM, Boehm FM. Prolonged end-stage fetal heart rate deceleration: A reanalysis. Obstet Gynecol 1981; 57:589–593.

**17.** Hon EH, Quilligan EJ. The classification of fetal heart rate. Conn Med 1967; 31:779–784.

**18.** Hon EH, Quilligan EJ. Electronic evaluation of fetal heart rate. Clin Obstet Gynecol 1968; 11:145–167.

**19.** Ingemarsson E, Ingemarsson I, Solum T, Westgren M. Influence of occiput posterior position on the fetal heart rate pattern. Obstet Gynecol 1980; 55:301–304.

**20.** Kero P, Antila K, Ylitalo V. Decreased heart rate variation in decerebration syndrome: Quantitative clinical criterion of brain death? Pediatrics 1978; 62:307–310.

**21.** Kitney RI, Rompelman O. The Study of Heart-Rate Variability. Clarendon Press, Oxford, England; 1980.

**22.** Knopf K, Parer JT, Espinoza ME, et al. Comparison of mathematical indices of fetal heart rate variability with visual assessment in the human and sheep. J Dev Physiol 1991; 16:367–372.

**23.** Koh KS, Cole TL, Orkin AJ. Listeria amnionitis as a cause of fetal distress. Am J Obstet Gynecol 1980; 136:261–263.

**24.** Krebs HB, Petres RE, Dunn LJ, Jordaan HVF, Segreti A. Intrapartum fetal heart rate monitoring. I. Classification and prognosis of fetal heart rate patterns. Am J Obstet Gynecol 1979; 133:762–772.

**25.** Krebs HB, Petres RE, Dunn LJ, Smith PJ. Intrapartum fetal heart rate monitoring VI. Prognostic significance of accelerations. Am J Obstet Gynecol 1982; 142:297–305.

**26.** Kubli FW, Hon EH, Khazin AF, Takemura H. Observations on heart rate and pH in the human fetus during labor. Am J Obstet Gynecol 1969; 104:1190–1206.

**27.** Martin CB Jr, DeHann J, van der Wildt B, et al. Mechanisms of late decelerations in the fetal heart rate. A study with autonomic blocking agents in fetal lambs. Europ J Obstet Gynecol Repro Biol 1979; 9:361–373.

**28.** Milio LA, Arnold SA, Parer JT. The relationship between fetal heart rate variability and hematocrit in Rh isoimmunization. Abstracts of Scientific Papers, 8th Annual Meeting of the Society for Perinatal Obstetricians, Las Vegas, 1988.

**29.** Miyazaki FS, Nevarez F. Saline amnioinfusion for relief of repetitive variable decelerations: A prospective randomized study. Am J Obstet Gynecol 1985; 153:301–306.

**30.** Murata Y, Martin CB, Ikenoue T, et al. Fetal heart rate accelerations and late decelerations during the course of intrauterine death in chronically catheterized rhesus monkeys. Am J Obstet Gynecol 1982; 144:218–223.

**31.** Murata Y, Miyake Y, Yamamoto T, et al. Experimentally produced sinusoidal fetal heart rate patterns in the chronically instrumented fetal lamb. Am J Obstet Gynecol 1985; 153:693–702.

**32.** Nathanielsz PW, Bailey A, Poore ER, et al. The relationship between myometrial activity and sleep state and breathing in fetal sheep throughout the last third of gestation. Am J Obstet Gynecol 1980; 138:653–659.

**33.** National Institutes of Health Research Planning Workshop. Electronic fetal heart rate monitoring: Research guidelines for interpretation. Am J Obstet Gynecol, in press, 1997.

**34.** Nijhuis JG, Crevels AJ, Van Dongen PWJ. Fetal brain death: The definition of a fetal heart rate pattern and its clinical consequences. Obstetrical and Gynecological Survey 1990; 45:229–232.

**35.** Nijhuis JC, Prechtl HFR, Martin CV Jr., Bots RSGM. Are there behavioural states in the human fetus? Early Hum Dev 1982; 6:177–195.

**36.** Parer JT. Fetal heart rate. In Creasy R, Resnick R, eds. Maternal-Fetal Medicine: Principles and Practice. 3rd ed. W.B. Saunders, Philadelphia, 1994, pp. 298–325.

**37.** Parer JT, Krueger TR, Harris JL. Fetal oxygen consumption and mechanisms of heart rate response during artificially produced late decelerations of fetal heart rate in sheep. Am J Obstet Gynecol 1980; 136:478–482.

**38.** Parer JT, Laros RK, Heilbron DC, Krueger TR. The roles of parasympathetic and beta-adrenergic activity in beat-to-beat fetal heart rate variability. In Kovach AGB, Monos E, Rubanyi G, eds. Cardiovascular Physiology-Heart, Peripheral Circulation & Methodology: Proceedings of the 28th International Congress of Physiological Sciences, Budapest, 1980 (Adv Phys Sci 1981; 8:327–329).

**39.** Parer WJ, Parer JT, Holbrook RH, Block BSB. Validity of mathematical methods of quantitating fetal heart rate variability. Am J Obstet Gynecol 1985; 153:402–409.

**40.** Paul RH, Suidan AK, Yeh S, et al. Clinical fetal monitoring. VII. The evaluation and significance of intrapartum baseline FHR variability. Am J Obstet Gynecol 1975; 123:206–210.

**41.** Phelan JP, Ahn MO. Perinatal observations in forty-eight neurologically impaired term infants. Am J Obstet Gynecol 1994; 171:424–431.

**42.** Porto M, Murata Y, Keegan KA, et al. Intermittent sinusoidal fetal heart rate: A sign of moderate fetal anemia. (In press) 1997.

**43.** Ralston DH, Shnider SM. The fetal and neonatal effects of regional anesthesia in obstetrics. Anesthesiology 1978; 48:34.

**44.** Rochard F, Schifrin BS, Goupil F, et al. Nonstressed fetal heart rate monitoring in the antepartum period. Am J Obstet Gynecol 1976; 126:699–706.

**45.** Schifrin BS, Dame L. Fetal heart rate patterns: Prediction of Apgar score. JAMA 1972; 219:1322–1326.

**46.** Schifrin BS, Hamilton-Rubinstein T, Shields JR. Fetal heart rate patterns and the timing of fetal injury. J Perinatol 1994; 14:174–181.

**47.** Silverman NH, Schmidt KG. Ultrasound evaluation of the fetal heart in Ultrasonography in Obstetrics and Gynecology. In Callen PW, ed. W.B. Saunders, Philadelphia, 1994, pp. 291–332.

**48.** Strong TH, Hetzler G, Sarno AP, Paul RH. Prophylactic intrapartum amnioinfusion: A randomized clinical trial. Am J Obstet Gynecol 1990; 162:1370–1375.

**49.** Zanini B, Paul RH, Huey JR. Intrapartum fetal heart rate: Correlation with scalp pH in the preterm fetus. Am J Obstet Gynecol 1980; 136:43–47.

# ■ *Chapter Ten*

# Asphyxia and Brain Damage

Fetal cerebral metabolism has been described in Chapter 5, together with many of the factors affecting it, particularly under conditions of limited oxygen availability. Most of the data were obtained from experimental animals, because for obvious reasons extensive instrumentation and experimental manipulation cannot be done in humans. Nevertheless, there is a large body of data in the human about asphyxial brain damage.

In this chapter we will examine two important clinical areas:

1. What do we know about the degree and duration of asphyxia which is sufficient to cause neuronal damage, and subsequent neuronal deficits?

2. What do we know about clinical recognition of this "intolerable" fetal asphyxia?

The importance of these two factors is obvious, and lies at the heart of conservative but realistic interpretation of fetal heart rate (FHR) patterns, and their rational management, based on currently available information and theory regarding the etiology of patterns. Thus timely recognition of the deteriorating (from the oxygenation point of view) fetus will limit its exposure to asphyxia, and continued observation of the fetus that is not deeply asphyxiated, but merely undergoing asphyxial stress, may avoid unnecessary cesarean section or other interventive delivery.

## I  ASPHYXIA AND FETAL MORBIDITY

The magnitude of the problem of fetal asphyxial damage is given in Table 10–1. Cerebral palsy (CP) is seen in approximately 2 to 3 per 1000 infants, and

**197**

**TABLE 10–1.   Newborn Outcome and Fetal Heart Rate Monitoring**

| | | |
|---|---|---|
| Long-term outcome | Cerebral palsy | 2.5 per 1000 |
| | Cerebral palsy due to intrapartum asphyxia | 0.25 per 1000 |
| Immediate newborn (NB) outcome | Umbilical artery pH ≤7 | 3.4 per 1000 |
| | NB seizures | 3.1 per 1000 |
| Intrapartum FHR | Variant ("abnormal") patterns | 300 per 1000 |
| | Variant patterns with reduced FHR variability | 30 per 1000 |

most estimates place the magnitude of CP due to intrapartum asphyxia at 10 percent or less of this total.[1, 18]

Newborn acidosis of pH 7.0 or less in the umbilical artery occurs in about 3 to 4 per 1000,[9] and newborn seizures are seen in about 3.1 per 1000,[25] although not all newborn seizures are due to asphyxia. These figures suggest that over 90 percent of babies with such severe acidosis, or with seizures at birth, will subsequently be normal. Nevertheless, these can be considered immediate outcomes that one would "prefer to avoid." The "overprediction" of fetal morbidity from FHR deceleration patterns is even more striking, as such patterns are 100-fold more common than severe acidosis, and 1000-fold more common than intrapartum asphyxia as a cause of cerebral palsy. Even FHR patterns with diminished or absent variability overcall immediate morbidity by 10-fold. By apparently pure coincidence, the number of stillbirths ascribed to asphyxia/hypoxia in 1985 in the United States was 1100,[26] or an incidence of 0.28 per 1000, about the same as the rate of CP attributed to intrapartum asphyxia.

*Asphyxia* has the pathologic meaning of insufficiency or absence of exchange of the respiratory gases, although etymologically it comes from the Greek, meaning pulseless. Its severity is described in terms of acidosis, hypoxemia, and hypercarbia. With prolonged hypoxia, anaerobic metabolism within the organism results in a lactic acidemia, which aggravates the acidosis (Table 10–2).

Fetal asphyxia almost always occurs as a result of insufficient umbilical or insufficient uterine blood flow. While this definition begs the question of what is "insufficient," it is recognized that reduction of these blood flows below a certain level will result in reduction of oxygen delivery to the fetus, and potentially to the brain, and this could result in reduced oxygen consumption by that organ. Under these conditions anaerobic metabolism may be utilized for high energy bond production, and lactate will be the end product. This will produce a metabolic acidosis in the tissue. At the same time there may be insufficient removal of carbon dioxide from the tissues, and a concomitant respiratory acidosis will develop.

There is little information on the rate of change of acid-base factors during asphyxia. Data from a single monkey fetus subjected to total oxygen deprivation at birth by cesarean section was presented by Myers et al.[17] Blood was sampled for 13 minutes from the femoral artery through a catheter placed before birth. The pH fell at 0.04 units/min, the carbon dioxide tension increased 6 mmHg/min, and the base excess fell slightly more than 1 mEq $\cdot$ L$^{-1}$/min. The oxygen tension fell to about 6 mmHg in about 2 minutes, and stabilized at that level. Sudden cessation of oxygen delivery to the fetus as a cause of asphyxia is probably clinically rare, with most cases of fetal asphyxia occurring by a reduction of gas exchange for a variable period of time. Obviously the rate of change of acid-base features and blood gases will likely differ in each fetus because of these variables.

It is obvious that asphyxia is not a sudden state of being, but rather represents a continuum of insufficiency of exchange of the respiratory gases (Table 10–3). This continuum begins as a "physiologic asphyxia" or acidemia when we consider the mild mixed metabolic and respiratory acidosis in umbilical cord blood specimens at the time of delivery in essentially all fetuses. Typical mean normal values are pH 7.27 (2.5th centile 7.10), carbon dioxide tension 52 (97.5th centile 74) mmHg, and base excess −4 (2.5th centile −11) mEq $\cdot$ L$^{-1}$.[9] The other end of the spectrum is the extremely severe metabolic and respiratory acidosis seen in babies suffering asphyxial brain damage following a catastrophic event such as a compressed prolapsed cord or complete abruption. In the latter case values may be of the order of pH 6.80, carbon dioxide tension 90 mmHg, and base excess −20 mEq $\cdot$ L$^{-1}$.[6]

In view of the fact that the state of asphyxia spans a continuum from "physiologic" to "terminal," and that pathologic results such as brain damage or death have not been rigidly defined in terms of acid-base state, it is not yet possible to assign any particular value or set of values to the term *asphyxia*. The duration and extent of metabolic acidosis and hypoxia that will result in neurologic damage to the human fetus are not known, and that is probably because there is an extremely wide variation of severity and duration of asphyxia that ultimately results in damage. The reason for this variation is

**TABLE 10–2.    The Consequences of Insufficiency of Exchange of Respiratory Gases**

| Insufficient → oxygen | Increased → lactate | Decreased HCO3$^-$ | —Metabolic acidosis | ⎫ |
| --- | --- | --- | --- | --- |
| Elevated carbon dioxide | | | —Respiratory acidosis | ⎬ Reduced pH ⎭ |

**TABLE 10–3.  Examples of Umbilical Cord Arterial Blood Gases and Acid-Base State in the Continuum of Hypoxemia, Hypercarbia, and Acidosis**

Average cord values at birth: "physiologic" asphyxia (e.g., pH 7.27, carbon dioxide tension 52 mmHg, base excess $-4$ mEq $\cdot$ L$^{-1}$)

Cord values associated with a risk of asphyxial neuronal death: "pathologic" asphyxia (e.g., pH 6.80, carbon dioxide tension 90 mmHg, base excess $-20$ mEq $\cdot$ L$^{-1}$)

probably because in any particular fetus, a number of other factors may be involved, such as stage of fetal development, metabolic state (e.g., carbohydrate reserves), and repetitiveness of asphyxial insults.[4]

The definition of asphyxia thus includes a reduction in oxygen content, an elevation of carbon dioxide tension, and a reduced pH. The definition of *insufficiency* can depend on arbitrary values of these three variables (e.g., mean $\pm$ 1 SD), or it may depend on a measurement of oxygen consumption falling significantly below the mean "normal" value (see Fig. 5–4). None of these criteria are particularly valuable for defining when there is permanent loss of function. An approach taken by Low and coworkers[15] was the combination of severity and duration resulting in motor and cognitive defects in approximately 50 percent of children; they defined this as an episode of hypoxia in excess of 1 hour resulting in a metabolic acidosis of the order of 25 mEq $\cdot$ L$^{-1}$ (defined by buffer base) and a pH less than 7.0. This buffer base value is approximately equal to a base excess of $-20$ mEq $\cdot$ L$^{-1}$. Other workers have used threshold values. Gilstrap et al.[3] suggested that newborns are at low risk for immediate complications resulting from intrapartum asphyxia unless the umbilical artery pH is less than 7 and Apgar scores are 3 or less at both 1 minute and 5 minutes. Goodwin and coworkers[6] reviewed the course of 129 term nonanomalous singleton infants with umbilical arterial pH below 7. They concluded that a pH below 6.8 with marked hypercarbia (carbon dioxide tension usually above 100 mmHg) and metabolic acidosis (base excess usually below $-15$ mEq $\cdot$ L$^{-1}$) relates best to neonatal death or major neurologic dysfunction. Goldaber et al.[5] defined a *pathologic fetal acidemia* as less than 7 in umbilical arterial blood in their review of 3506 term newborns with an umbilical arterial pH of less than 7.20.

These are appropriate approaches to the problem but undoubtedly are of limited predictive utility. We therefore believe that the term *asphyxia* should not be used to denote a specific pathologic state but rather should be used to define simply what it is, that is, elevated carbon dioxide and reduced oxygen, with a metabolic component. The term *asphyxia* should simply be used as a preceding descriptor for the acid-base features of umbilical arterial blood and the weakness of these values as a predictor of fetal damage should be implied.

Despite these limitations of definition, it is of value to examine fetal responses to asphyxia in order to determine compensatory mechanisms.

## FETAL HEART RATE MONITORING AND OUTCOME

### A  Can Intolerable Fetal Asphyxia Be Recognized?

Interpretation of FHR monitoring patterns is in an extraordinarily confused state in North America, and there is great variation in opinions with regard to what is "abnormal." There is no argument anymore about the fact that many babies exhibiting various types of decelerations will *not* be born asphyxiated, yet many people persist in calling such patterns *abnormal* or some other similar qualitative terms such as *nonreassuring* or *ominous.* These terms have limited usefulness and we believe that they should be replaced by other more descriptive terms.

There is general agreement amongst essentially all clinicians that the baby with a heart rate in the "normal" range, that is, 110 to 160 beats/min, with normal FHR variability, that is, an amplitude range of 6 beats/min or greater, and absent decelerations is essentially always nonasphyxiated. Therefore, it seems reasonable to refer to this pattern as the "normal" FHR pattern.

There is also general agreement that the fetus with absent FHR variability, a heart rate within or outside the normal range, and deep variable or late decelerations, is presumed to be asphyxiated, and expeditious delivery is indicated (see Figs. 9–12 and 9–14). The same is true of a deep persistent bradycardia, for example, 60 beats/min or less, with absent variability (in the absence of congenital heart block). Clinically this also represents a fetus with presumed asphyxia and expeditious delivery is indicated (see Fig. 11–3).

Between these two extremes, that is, the normal and the presumed asphyxiated baby, there exists a vast array of FHR patterns which fit neither of these fairly accurate predictions. Thus, the fetus with normal FHR variability, even in the face of reflex late decelerations or variable decelerations, is almost invariably born nonasphyxiated and vigorous. Such babies should be described as having "variant" FHR patterns rather than "abnormal" FHR patterns. It is inappropriate to label such patterns "fetal distress" because such babies are not asphyxiated, although they may have mild elevations of carbon dioxide and mild depressions of base excess as a result of a cumulative mild reduction in exchange of the respiratory gases. Appropriate management for such fetuses is an attempt to abolish the decelerations, or, if unsuccessful, then observation of the evolution of the pattern to be sure that a cumulative asphyxia does not develop resulting in fetal decompensation. This is currently noted by continued retention of normal FHR variability. Should FHR variability decrease to the point where it can be predicted to result in asphyxial decompensation before a vaginal delivery, then this can be labeled "fetal intolerance of labor." This then would be an appropriate indication for operative delivery.

The prognostic capacity of FHR variability has been the subject of much discussion. It was commonly stated in the past that FHR monitoring is extremely accurate in diagnosing fetal vigor when the pattern is normal, but that it is poor for determining depression when the pattern is "abnormal."[10, 24] That is, its specificity, or ability to correctly diagnose "normal," was thought to be poor. This resulted in the overdiagnosis of "fetal distress," and at times unnecessary intervention leading to either cesarean section or potentially traumatic operative vaginal deliveries. This may be true if one interprets FHR patterns according to older concepts which considered the prominent "abnormality" to be decelerations of FHR with contractions.

Empirical clinical evidence strongly suggests that the addition of the determination of FHR variability to the FHR pattern interpretation can aid in improving specificity. Evidence for this view has taken the form of clinical observations[2] or retrospective surveys of outcome following monitoring.[7, 13, 23] The common trend in these studies is that the presence of FHR variability is almost invariably associated with fetal vigor at birth, even in the presence of various decelerations or bradycardias. A further observation is that of babies which died in utero while being monitored, none had the presence of normal FHR variability.[20] The corollary of this observation is that if the FHR has normal variability, the fetus is at low risk for immediate death due to asphyxia. The preceding observations and widespread clinical experience have resulted in the acceptance of FHR variability by many clinicians as a prime indicator of fetal vigor.[21]

The acceptance of the efficacy of this approach to FHR interpretation is not, however, universal,[8, 14, 16] and we believe that the overdiagnosis of the "asphyxiated" fetus will continue until a physiologic basis for FHR variability is demonstrated, leading to more rational interpretation. The original interpretation of FHR patterns stressed the decelerations (late or variable decelerations) occurring with contractions, and equated their presence to "fetal distress," which then dictated operative intervention.[11] The alternative interpretation states that the decelerations, or bradycardias, indicate intermittent asphyxial "stresses" (generally insufficiency of uterine or umbilical blood flow), while the collective influence of these stresses on the fetal physiologic compensatory mechanisms is determined by the decrease or loss of FHR variability, signifying a cumulative oxygen debt and decompensation.[21] Thus the presence of FHR variability indicates central (nervous system and/or myocardial) normoxia, while its decrease in the presence of the stress patterns indicates a decrease in the oxygenation of these organs.

The source of FHR variability is clearly complex, with inputs from many cycling physiologic phenomena, including respiratory arrhythmia, blood pressure fluctuations, and thermoregulation, at least in the adult. However, many of the observations are most consistent with the theory that the presence of normal variability requires integrity of the variability pathways of (a) the cerebral cortex, (b) the midbrain, (c) the vagus nerve, and (d) the cardiac conduction system (see Chapter 9).

As noted earlier, it has long been recognized that FHR variability can be affected by numerous influences besides asphyxia. Such influences include congenital anomalies and drugs, and in some cases there is no apparent cause, although the baby is normal at birth. Examples of some factors responsible for decreased or absent variability include anencephaly, complete heart block, narcotic administration (presumably acting on the central nervous system), and atropine administration (presumably blocking oscillatory influences transmitted by the vagus nerve). Variability is also affected by changes in fetal state.

It is important to be aware of such factors in order to make the appropriate distinction between asphyxial and nonasphyxial causes of decreased variability.

## B  Clinical Implications

There are basically three common means by which the human fetus can become asphyxiated or hypoxic (Table 10–4): (a) insufficiency of uterine blood flow,[27] (b) insufficiency of umbilical blood flow,[12] or (c) a decrease in maternal arterial oxygen content.[19] Other mechanisms, such as fetal anemia or increased fetal oxygen needs (in pyrexia), are relatively rarely seen clinically (see Chapters 3 and 4).

In clinical obstetrics these three common mechanisms can be recognized during labor (that is, in the presence of uterine contractions) by various FHR

---

**TABLE 10–4.  Causes of Fetal Hypoxia/Asphyxia**

**Major**
   Inadequate uterine blood flow
   Inadequate umbilical blood flow
   Inadequate maternal arterial oxygen

**Rare**
   Increased fetal oxygen needs (e.g., fever)
   Fetal anemia (e.g., hemolytic diseases, or fetal–maternal bleeding)

patterns. Uterine contractions are thought to cause the transient decelerations because of the concomitant decrease in uterine blood flow with the contraction,[11] or an associated decrease in umbilical blood flow (e.g., due to umbilical cord compression).[11] The patterns corresponding to the above mechanisms are (a) late decelerations, (b) variable decelerations, and (c) persistent fetal bradycardia (see Chapter 9). A prolonged stepwise insufficiency of uterine or umbilical blood flow would likewise be recognized as a bradycardia. It has been proposed that a fetus with normal FHR variability will not revert to one with absent FHR variability caused by asphyxia during labor unless one of these asphyxial "stress" patterns is present[21] (Table 10–5). On the other hand, if the FHR variability is absent on initial application of the FHR monitor, then it may not be possible to distinguish between asphyxial and nonasphyxial causes of decreased FHR variability, and the fetal stimulation test or fetal blood sampling for determination of acid-base status may need to be carried out (see Chapter 12).

The clinical means by which we currently use the above definition to ensure adequate fetal compensation is by noting the progress of severity of the FHR stress patterns, and the retention of FHR variability. Intermittent or sustained decreases in FHR variability in the presence of stress patterns are assumed to signal the onset of decompensation, unless asphyxia is ruled out by ancillary testing, such as stimulation testing or fetal blood sampling. It is hoped that future physiologic studies, and correlation with FHR patterns, will further refine the definition of "fetal distress" and make the diagnosis more accurate in the clinical setting.

## C  What Is Fetal Distress?

The concept of "fetal distress" has been discussed previously,[22] as well as the fact that the term is so ill-defined and loosely used that it has lost its usefulness. An appropriate, though awkward, definition of fetal distress is *progressive persistent asphyxia of such severity that if it is not relieved will result in (a) breakdown of the compensatory fetal blood flow redistribution, (b) reduced cerebral metabolism, and (c) neuronal cell death.*

It is currently widely accepted that this cardiorespiratory decompensation can be clinically noted during labor by reduced or absent FHR variability in the appropriate setting, that is, in the setting of severe variable or late decelerations, or a bradycardia.

**TABLE 10–5.  The Central Dogma**

Decreasing FHR variability due to asphyxia during labor occurs after some substantial asphyxial stress, which will be manifest as decelerations (usually severe variable or late) or a bradycardia

**TABLE 10–6.  Factors Consistent with a Diagnosis of Intrapartum Asphyxial Brain Damage**

FHR pattern with absent variability at birth
Umbilical artery pH <7.0 (more convincing if <6.8)
Umbilical artery base excess $<-15\ mEq \cdot L^{-1}$ (more convincing if $<-20$)
Apgar score <3 at 5 min (more convincing if still <3 at 10 min)
Neurologic signs in newborn (more convincing if seizures)
Multiorgan damage in newborn (renal, heart, etc.)

In specific cases the term *fetal distress* can be replaced by more descriptive terms such as "presumed fetal asphyxia" or "fetal intolerance of labor," together with a full description of the FHR pattern, including time trends.

# D  Diagnosis of Intrapartum Asphyxial Brain Damage

We are now at the point where we can list the features which are needed to confirm a diagnosis of intrapartum fetal asphyxia lasting until the moment of birth as a cause of subsequent neurologic morbidity (Table 10–6). It is not always possible to find all six items in any particular case, but some factors (e.g., a severe metabolic acidosis and low Apgar score) must be present to support the diagnosis. An important observation is that even the presence of all of these factors does not confirm that brain damage will occur. Also, an abnormal outcome may be due to a different cause occurring concomitantly (e.g., a developmental abnormality) with intrapartum asphyxia. Such a view is supported by the catch phrase "does brain damage cause intrapartum asphyxia?" Thus, a fetus with a prior episode of damage due to hypoxia-ischemia, a toxin or infection, may have myocardial or other damage which predisposes it to cardiorespiratory decomposition during labor.

# REFERENCES

1. Blair E, Stanley FJ. Intrapartum asphyxia: A rare cause of cerebral palsy. J Pediatr 1988; 112:515–519.
2. Boehm FH. FHR variability: key to fetal well-being. Contemp Obstet Gynecol 1977; 9:57–68.
3. Gilstrap LC, Leveno JK, Burns J, et al. Diagnosis of birth asphyxia on the basis of fetal pH, Apgar score, and newborn cerebral dysfunction. Am J Obstet Gynecol 1989; 161:825–830.
4. Gluckman PD, Williams CE. When and why do brain cells die? Dev Med Child Neurol 1992; 34:1010–1021.
5. Goldaber KG, Gilstrap LC, Leveno KJ, et al. Pathologic fetal acidemia. Obstet Gynecol 1991; 78:1103–1108.

6. Goodwin TM, Belai I, Hernandez P, et al. Asphyxial complications in the term newborn with severe umbilical acidemia. Am J Obstet Gynecol 1992; 162:1506–1512.

7. Hammacher K, Huter KA, Bokelmann J, Werners PH. Foetal heart frequency and perinatal condition of foetus and newborn. Gynaecologia (Basel) 1968; 166:348–360.

8. Haverkamp AD, Orleans M, Langendoerfer S, et al. A controlled trial of the differential effects of intrapartum fetal monitoring. Am J Obstet Gynecol 1979; 134:399–408.

9. Helwig Jane T, Parer JT, Kilpatrick SJ, Laros RK Jr. Umbilical cord blood acid-base state: What is normal? Am J Obstet Gynecol 1996; 174:1807-1814.

10. Hon EH. Detection of fetal distress. In Wood C, ed. Proceedings of the Fifth World Congress of Gynecology and Obstetrics. Butterworth, Melbourne, 1967.

11. Hon EH. An Atlas of Fetal Heart Rate Patterns. Harty Press, New Haven, Conn, 1968.

12. Itskovitz J, LaGamma EF, Rudolph AM. The effect of reducing umbilical blood flow on fetal oxygenation. Am J Obstet Gynecol 1983; 145:813–818.

13. Krebs HB, Petres RE, Dunn LJ, et al. Intrapartum fetal heart rate monitoring: I. Classification and prognosis of fetal heart rate patterns. Am J Obstet Gynecol 1979; 133:762–772.

14. Leveno KJ, Cunningham FS, Nelson S, et al. A prospective comparison of selective and universal electronic monitoring in 34,995 pregnancies. N Engl J Med 1986; 315:615–619.

15. Low JA, Galbraith RS, Muir DW, et al. Factors associated with motor and cognitive deficits in children after intrapartum fetal hypoxia. Am J Obstet Gynecol 1984; 148:533.

16. MacDonald D, Grant A, Sheridan-Pereira M, et al. The Dublin randomized controlled trial of intrapartum fetal heart rate monitoring. Am J Obstet Gynecol 1985; 152:524–539.

17. Myers RE. Two patterns of perinatal brain damage and their conditions of occurrence. Am J Obstet Gynecol 1972; 112:246–276.

18. Nelson KB, Ellenberg JH. Antecedents of cerebral palsy. N Engl J Med 1986; 315:81–86.

19. Parer JT. The effect of acute maternal hypoxia on fetal oxygenation and the umbilical circulation in the sheep. Eur J Obstet Gynecol Reprod Biol 1980; 10:125–136.

20. Parer JT. Handbook of Fetal Heart Rate Monitoring. W.B. Saunders, Philadelphia, 1983.

21. Parer JT. Fetal heart rate. In Creasy R, Resnik R, eds. Maternal-Fetal Medicine: Principles and Practice. 3rd ed. W.B. Saunders, Philadelphia, 1994, pp. 298–325.

22. Parer JT, Livingstone EG. What is fetal distress? Am J Obstet Gynecol 1990; 162:1421–1427.

23. Paul RH, Suidan AK, Yeh S, et al. Clinical fetal monitoring: VII. The evaluation and significance of intrapartum baseline FHR variability. Am J Obstet Gynecol 1975; 123:206–210.

24. Schifrin BS, Dame L. Fetal heart rate patterns: prediction of Apgar score. JAMA 1972; 219:1322–1325.

25. Thacker SB, Stroup DF, Peterson HB. Efficacy and safety of intrapartum electronic fetal monitoring: An update. Obstet Gynecol 1995; 86:613–620.

26. United States Preventive Services Task Force. Guide to Clinical Preventive Services, 1989.

27. Yaffe H, Parer JT, Block BS, Llanos AJ. Cardiorespiratory responses to graded reductions in uterinblood flow in the sheep fetus. J Dev Physiol 1987; 9:325–336.

# Part Five

# CLINICAL MANAGEMENT

# ■ *Chapter Eleven*

# Management of Variant Patterns

## I CLINICAL MANAGEMENT

Over the 30 or so years since the introduction of continuous fetal heart rate (FHR) monitoring, there have been numerous recommendations for action based on certain patterns. Algorithms, some more complete than others, can be found in a number of the publications referred to in Chapters 10 and 15. Because of their wide variation, they will not be reviewed here. In general there has been an evolution and maturing of these protocols over time, particularly recognizing the fact that up to one in three babies has a variant (formerly called "abnormal" or "ominous") pattern but this is many times higher than the incidence of severe acidosis, or seizures, or cerebral palsy (see Chapter 10). Thus dramatic intervention is in fact rarely required in such patterns to avoid damaging fetal asphyxia.

In this chapter we present an approach to management which attempts to give guidance for avoiding the rare case of asphyxial damage in a timely manner, and restricting potentially hazardous intervention (i.e., cesarean section or vaginal operative delivery) to appropriate cases.

## A The Decision-Making Process

It is important to recognize that decisions and diagnoses of the state of fetal oxygenation during labor in the presence or variant patterns are rarely static, but changing over time. Also decisions are made in the light of the clinical situation (e.g., presence of prematurity, intrauterine growth retardation, thick meconium, clinical abruption).

**209**

A series of diagnoses based on the FHR patterns can be developed, and one such schema is shown in Table 11–1. This is a personal protocol, and it has not been subjected to a rigorous trial, so it is based on imperfect information which eventually must be confirmed or refuted. However, the same limitations are true of all published management recommendations and algorithms. The tabulation presented here has the benefit of at least a partial physiologic basis, and has performed well in empirical usage.

The five diagnoses recognize the fact that there is an evolution of patterns from that signifying normal fetal oxygenation, diagnosis no. 1, to that which is highly predictive of actual or impending damaging asphyxia, diagnosis no. 5. This is somewhat similar to the five action scores used by Keith et al.[1] in the development of an expert computerized management schema. It is believed to be more realistic than the simple categorization of patterns as "reassuring" versus "nonreassuring" used by some clinicians. In addition, this schema avoids the pejorative label of "abnormal FHR patterns," which in the past has been applied to every variation from the average value of the baseline rate, or variability, or the presence of any periodic or episodic changes. As noted above we prefer the term *variant pattern* for these latter patterns.

The five diagnoses are accompanied by a description of the FHR patterns leading to the diagnoses, and recommended action (Table 11–2). The schema is unlikely to be all inclusive for all patterns which are likely to be encountered. Babies will likely change diagnostic number in relation to progress in labor, or results of in utero treatment, so the diagnosis could conceivably change even over a 10-minute period. Note that diagnosis is easiest if the baby begins with a normal FHR pattern (i.e., diagnosis no. 1) and the pattern evolves progressively through to the higher numbers. Diagnosis can be more difficult if the initial FHR tracing encountered is one of the higher numbers, and one does not have the benefit of evolution being observed. Some of the dilemmas in this situation are addressed in Chapter 12.

Enlargement on the various diagnoses, FHR patterns, and clinical action will be found in the following sections, where each of the major patterns signifying or resulting in fetal oxygen insufficiency (or reductions below average levels) are discussed.

**TABLE 11–1.    The Spectrum of Fetal Heart Rate Diagnoses Signifying the State of Fetal Oxygenation**

1. The baby is well oxygenated.
2. The baby is still well oxygenated centrally.
3. The baby is still well oxygenated centrally, but the FHR pattern suggests reductions in oxygen which may result in accumulation of fetal oxygen debt.
4. The baby may be on the verge of decompensation.
5. The baby has evidence of actual or impending damaging asphyxia.

**TABLE 11–2.  Fetal Diagnosis Based on Fetal Heart Rate Pattern, and Action to Avert or Minimize Asphyxial Damage**

| Diagnosis | FHR Pattern | Action |
|---|---|---|
| The baby is well oxygenated | Normal rate, normal FHRV, ± accelerations, no periodic or episodic decelerations | None |
| The baby is still well oxygenated centrally | Normal FHRV, ± accelerations, mild variant pattern (i.e., bradycardia, LD, VD) | Conservative in utero therapy; expect abolition of variant pattern if cause reversed |
| The baby is still well oxygenated centrally, but the FHR pattern suggests reductions in oxygen which may result in accumulation of fetal oxygen debt | Normal FHRV, ± accelerations, moderate/severe variant pattern (i.e., bradycardia, LD, VD) | Continue conservative in utero therapy; ± amnioinfusion, ± stimulation testing; check ability to deliver rapidly in case pattern worsens |
| The baby may be on the verge of decompensation | Decreasing FHRV, ± accelerations, moderate/severe variant patterns (i.e., bradycardia, LD, VD) | Deliver if spontaneous delivery remote, or if ancillary testing (stimulation and/or blood sampling) supports diagnosis of decompensation; normal testing results may allow time to await a vaginal delivery |
| The baby has evidence of actual or impending damaging asphyxia | FHRV decreasing to undetectable, no accelerations, moderate/severe variant patterns (i.e., bradycardia, LD, VD) | Deliver; may attempt further evaluation or in utero therapy if it does not unduly delay delivery |

FHRV, fetal heart rate variability; LD, late decelerations; VD, variable decelerations.

# II  MANAGEMENT OF LATE DECELERATIONS

The definition, presumed etiology, and some aspects of management of late decelerations have been discussed in Chapter 9. In this chapter we will summarize our current approach.

If one examines any heart rate tracing it is almost always possible to find at least one deceleration which fits the criteria of late deceleration. However, because an essential part of the definition is that they are persistent, we will only consider here those that are either seen with every contraction, or come in runs or families of late decelerations (see Fig. 9–9).

Let us first consider late decelerations with normal FHR variability—reflex late decelerations. They can occur from first placement of the monitor, or may appear during the course of labor. They may be in response to lowered uterine blood flow due to a recognizable event, such as a slight drop in blood pressure following activation of a regional anesthetic, the onset of more frequent or stronger contractions, the gradual onset of hypovolemia, due to insufficient fluid intake in a laboring mother, or a relatively minor manifestation of the supine hypotensive syndrome.

In most of the above examples the decelerations can be abolished by the conservative means outlined in Chapter 8. As noted previously, attempts should be made to abolish the decelerations, because if they persist, and become more profound and prolonged, they may evolve into the nonreflex type, manifested by a reduction and finally loss of FHR variability. This latter pattern is assumed to represent asphyxial decompensation and is an indication for ancillary testing (see Chapter 8) or delivery.

The clinical observation has been made that the majority of term, normally grown fetuses will be able to tolerate at least 30 minutes of reflex late decelerations before decompensation, so this can be considered to be the time available for conservative management to abolish the decelerations, or, if they cannot be abolished, time to prepare for a possible operative delivery. The specific preparations to be made are dependent on the institution, its staffing, and its facilities, so no overall recommendations can be made for all cases.

There is an accepted evolution which occurs from reflex to nonreflex decelerations during labor (see Fig. 9–12). There is a gradual deepening of the decelerations, then the intermittent reduction of variability, and finally the loss of variability with persistence of the decelerations. It should be emphasized that this is a general rule which applies in specific circumstances, namely, a gradual rather than sudden decrease in maternal placental function (specifically a reduction in uterine blood flow, or oxygen flow), and the evolution from a normal pattern. There appear to be occasional exceptions to this pattern of evolution, although this is not well established. This may occur in some cases of chorioamnionitis, and possibly postmaturity syndrome. Cases have been noted where the evolution to reduced or absent FHR variability occurs with relatively minor late decelerations, and, in chorioamnionitis, a relatively mild tachycardia.

Nonreflex late decelerations (persistent late decelerations without FHR variability) which cannot be abolished are, we believe, an indication for delivery, unless ancillary testing can be done without unduly delaying delivery and the results rule out asphyxia (Fig. 11–1). We believe that the majority of fetuses with such late decelerations are either already asphyxiated, or will soon become so, and rapid delivery will minimize exposure of the fetus to such asphyxia. Admittedly, a small percentage may in fact not be deeply asphyxiated but may simply have reflex late decelerations accompanied by a nonasphyxial decrease in FHR variability. While this could be determined by ancillary testing, such as stimulation testing or fetal blood sampling, the relatively small number of institutions where fetal blood sampling is available motivates the recommendation for rapid delivery if there is no response to stimulation testing.

Why might a baby have reflex late decelerations with an accompanying nonasphyxial reduced variability? One possible reason is drugs (e.g., narcotics, sedatives, or magnesium sulfate), though our observations suggest that following these drugs it is rare to have a total loss of variability, and if the drug is given episodically rather than as an infusion, it is rare to have a persistent absence of variability.

A further reason for a nonasphyxial reduction of variability is a neurologic deficit, either developmental, or acquired due to a prior global or regional asphyxial or ischemic event. If the event is global asphyxia from which the fetus has subsequently recovered its oxygenation, there may be reduced or absent FHR variability without late decelerations, but if there is persistent cardiac hypoxia, there should be associated late decelerations (see Chapter 12). There is no simple rapid means of ruling in or out such prior damage in the majority of cases, without obtaining a high-quality ultrasound, and ancillary testing. Indeed such neurologic damage may not be diagnosable on ultrasound imaging.

A further observation is that despite late decelerations and absent FHR variability and in spite of the theoretical mechanisms of loss of variability noted above (see Chapters 9 and 10) there is no assurance that the baby will in fact have asphyxial neurologic damage (Fig. 11–1). Thus the recommendation for immediate delivery gives the baby the benefit of the uncertainty in diagnosis. Whether such a baby has in fact not suffered damage, or is able to recover from neuronal damage by remodeling, is unlikely to be known in any specific fetus, but must await future development.

## III   MANAGEMENT OF VARIABLE DECELERATIONS

The description and presumed etiology of variable decelerations has been given in Chapter 9. Variable decelerations may occur sporadically in the antepartum period, during the latent phase of labor, during the first stage

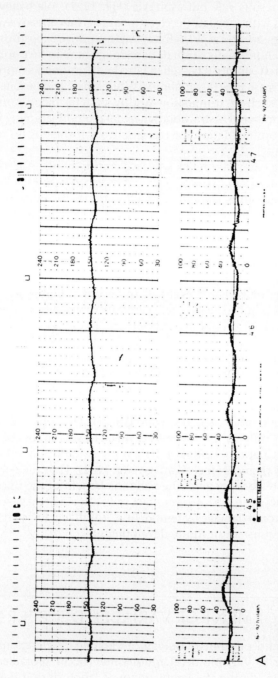

**FIGURE 11–1.**    (A) This term patient, with a normally grown baby, entered labor and delivery with the tracing shown.

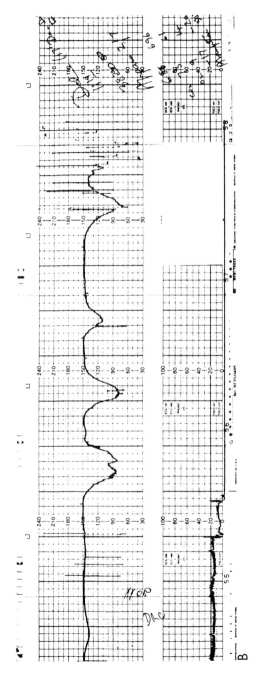

**FIGURE 11–1.** *Continued* (B) She was taken to the operating room, where membranes were ruptured and an internal electrode placed. This apparently stimulated further uterine activity, giving deeper late decelerations. At cesarean section a large placental abruption with a retroplacental clot was found. The umbilical arterial pH was 6.88, and base excess −17 mEq • L⁻¹. The Apgar scores were 2 (1 minute) and 7 (5 minutes). The child is developmentally normal at age 10.

active phase of labor, or during the second stage. As noted earlier the etiology may vary depending on when they occur.

We will first consider the management of variable decelerations occurring in the latent phase of labor, and we will further assume that they are occurring after a reactive admission FHR trace (nonreactive admission strips will be described in Chapter 12). These variable decelerations are usually of modest depth and duration, sometimes called the *mild–moderate category*. The assumption made when there are variable decelerations occurring with mild uterine activity early in labor is that they are probably due to cord compression. The usual approach is to attempt to modify the depth and duration of the decelerations or abolish them by altering the position of the mother, that is, to the lateral or other position. As noted earlier, it is extremely unlikely that a fetus will decompensate from the oxygenation point of view in the presence of such mild–moderate variable decelerations, but on the other hand they may develop into severe variable decelerations, which may eventually result in compromise. Therefore it is reasonable to attempt to abolish any such decelerations.

If the decelerations cannot be abolished by conservative means, and they become deeper and more prolonged, one may wish to obtain an ultrasound examination to determine the adequacy of amniotic fluid (see Chapter 2). If the amniotic fluid index is low this might well explain the decelerations, and amnioinfusion may be used to abolish them, although such an approach is by no means mandatory, and simply attempting position change is less interventive.

A similar management schema is acceptable for the first-stage active phase of labor in the presence of mild–moderate variable decelerations, and a reactive FHR tracing. That is, attempts should be made to abolish the decelerations by conservative means. Should they not be modified by position changes of the mother, then the patient may either be observed for progress of the decelerations, or amnioinfusion may be carried out if the amniotic fluid index is low.

If it is not possible to modify or abolish such variable decelerations, then no particular further management is necessary except to observe the decelerations for evolution to the more serious type. This implies continuous electronic monitoring, and the ability to intervene or react in a reasonable period of time if such an evolution occurs.

Should the variable decelerations evolve to the severe type, then fetal asphyxial decompensation becomes a possibility. The clinical observation has been made that such decompensation rarely occurs in less than 30 minutes in the normally grown, term fetus. Therefore, this time is available for planning potential intervention, which usually means cesarean section during the latent- or first-stage active phase.

During severe variable decelerations the heart rate pattern must be observed for an intermittent reduction in FHR variability during and following the variable deceleration (see Figs. 9–14 and 11–2). Should this begin to occur and still abolition of the decelerations cannot be achieved by the means outlined above, then delivery is recommended. Delivery is recommended before the total loss of variability because this may signify asphyxial decompensation, and indeed must be presumed to do so unless asphyxia can be ruled out by ancillary methods (see Chapter 8).

Severe variable decelerations in the presence of frequent uterine activity may become confluent and form a prolonged deceleration, and eventually a bradycardia. Therefore in the presence of persistent severe variable decelerations it is prudent to attempt to maintain uterine contractions more than 2 minutes apart. This may be achieved by turning down the oxytocin dosage (if it is being used), or use of the lateral position in the laboring mother, which sometimes results in spacing out of the contractions. Should the severe variable decelerations evolve to a bradycardia, then this is managed as described in the next section.

Variable decelerations in the second stage of labor are managed somewhat differently. As noted in Chapter 9, the incidence of variable decelerations increases in the second stage, and they are more likely to be caused by head compression (and subsequent dural stimulation) than cord compression. Intervention by an operative vaginal delivery can often be carried out safely, and in fact may well be elected by some practitioners rather than tolerating persistent severe variable decelerations. A fuller treatment of their management is outlined in Chapter 13.

## IV  MANAGEMENT OF BRADYCARDIAS

As described in Chapter 9, a bradycardia is here technically defined as a baseline heart rate below 110 beats/min with specific additional criteria. The general observation has been made that the lower the bradycardia, the more likely is the possibility of fetal compromise. A persistent heart rate below 60 beats/min without FHR variability (in the absence of heart block) is highly predictive of asphyxial compromise.

We will first treat management of bradycardias with the assumption that there is a normal FHR admission strip, that is, a normal rate with normal variability and absence of persistent decelerations. Should this tracing evolve into a bradycardia with a heart rate between 100 and 110 beats/min with normal variability, then this can probably be tolerated by most fetuses for essentially unlimited periods of time.

The same may well also be true of a bradycardia between 80 and 100 beats/min with normal variability, that is, there is no particular limit of time when this bradycardia will evolve into a decompensatory pattern, which would be signified by decrease and finally loss of FHR variability. Nevertheless,

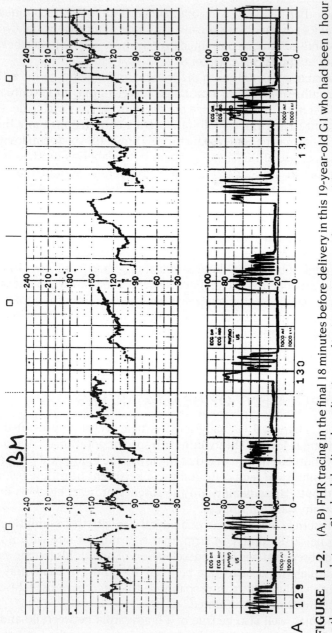

**FIGURE 11–2.** (A, B) FHR tracing in the final 18 minutes before delivery in this 19-year-old G1 who had been 1 hour in the second stage. She had declined medication and/or intervention, and was unable to control involuntary pushing. Note the evolution of this pattern from mild–moderate variable decelerations, to deeper variable decelerations, and finally to a loss of FHR variability. A tachycardia developed, though this is not invariably seen in such cases. The fetus was moderately depressed with a moderate metabolic acidosis, but was easily resuscitated and did well.

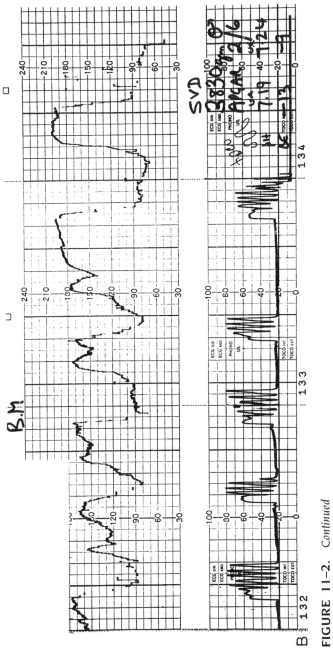

**FIGURE 11–2.**  *Continued*

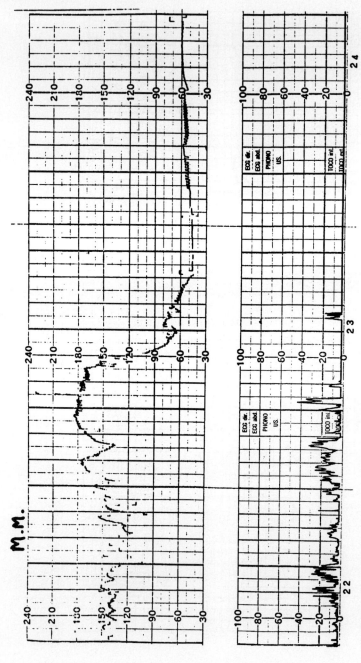

**FIGURE 11-3.** Sudden prolonged fetal bradycardia in a woman with a fatal amniotic fluid embolism early in labor. There is immediate bradycardia to less than 60 beats/min with the onset of maternal cyanosis and pulmonary edema. There is also loss of FHR variability. An asphyxiated baby was delivered by cesarean section approximately 20 minutes later.

most practitioners would make some preparations for an emergency delivery in case decompensation should occur, even though they may not carry out the emergency delivery should the pattern resolve.

When a persistent bradycardia occurs with a rate between 60 and 80 beats/min most practitioners attempt to abolish it, and if it cannot be rapidly abolished, make immediate preparation for delivery. Delivery under these conditions would be called for if the bradycardia does not resolve and the variability declines. However, in the presence of retained variability then observation is acceptable (see Fig. 9–20).

A persistent unresolvable heart rate below 60 beats/min in the absence of heart block is an obstetric emergency and delivery should be carried out, more emergently (if possible) in the absence of FHR variability (Fig. 11–3).

The management of bradycardias in the second stage is modified by the possibility of rapid emergency vaginal delivery, rather than cesarean section, so in general a bradycardia may be tolerated for a longer period than in the first stage (see Chapter 13).

## REFERENCE

**1.** Keith RDF, Beckley S, Garibaldi JM, et al. A multicentre comparative study of 17 experts and an intelligent computer system for managing labor using the cardiotocogram. Br J Obstet Gynaecol 1995; 102:688–700.

# ■ Chapter Twelve

# Initial Absent Fetal Heart Rate Variability

Every clinician has at one stage or another been faced with the fetus that enters labor and delivery with absent variability of the fetal heart rate (FHR), which does not resolve with the usual conservative means of optimizing uterine and umbilical blood flows and fetal oxygenation. In this chapter such cases are discussed, with the understanding that we do not yet have the complete solution to this often difficult management problem.

As noted numerous times in this manual, the presence of normal FHR variability signifies normal fetal oxygenation. However, the absence of FHR variability does not necessarily signify insufficient oxygenation, or damaging asphyxia. In specific settings, it can give rise to the diagnosis of "presumed fetal asphyxia," and trigger certain clinical action. An example of this would be decreasing and/or finally absent variability following the development of deepening and unremitting variable decelerations (see Fig. 9–14).

The absence of variability, in the absence of one of three patterns signifying a mechanism of insufficient oxygenation during labor, is a situation which presents great difficulty in management, primarily because the clinician lacks the assurance of normal oxygenation. The absence of the "appropriate setting" (i.e., the patterns noted above) is somewhat reassuring, but such cases usually cause concern to the delivery team.

---

## I  POSSIBLE NONASPHYXIAL DIAGNOSES WITH THE FLAT BASELINE DURING LABOR

### A  Quiet Sleep State
There is abundant evidence that FHR patterns vary depending on the fetal state [9] (see Fig. 2–1). Variability is evident and accelerations are frequent during

rapid eye movement (REM) sleep, and the amplitude of variability is substantially suppressed during quiet (non-REM) sleep. Variability and accelerations are maximal during "active wakefulness," such that the accelerations may become confluent, with a sustained high heart rate satisfying the criteria of tachycardia (see Chapter 9).

It is generally possible to distinguish the fetus undergoing quiet sleep by several observations. Firstly, the variability is usually reduced, rather than totally absent, although fetuses tend to have their own characteristic "quality" of variability, and some are quite flat during quiet sleep periods. The mean period of cycling between quiet and active sleep is about 20 minutes, so this, and the absence of periodic changes or bradycardia preceding the reduced variability, is usually diagnostic. The duration of the state can vary widely, however, and may sometimes last over an hour.

It is often possible to terminate a period of quiet sleep by stimulation of the fetus, either tactile (though this is not universally agreed upon) or vibroacoustic stimulation. This should provide reassurance in uncertain cases.

## B  Idiopathic

As noted earlier, the amount of FHR variability displayed by different fetuses varies, and it is reasonable to assume that some totally normal fetuses will have variability below our arbitrarily determined normal range. It is even likely that some normal fetuses have so little variability that it is visually undetectable. If this is so the incidence is probably quite low, because this category of "absent variability" is rare in various FHR pattern surveys, as also is the incidence of flat baselines due to asphyxia or other causes.

## C  Drugs

A number of drugs, particularly narcotics and tranquilizers, are known to reduce FHR variability. It is presumed that the action of the drugs is on the higher nervous centers. Magnesium sulfate, commonly used in preeclamptics and for treatment of preterm labor, also can cause a reduction in variability.

It is relatively unusual for such drugs to cause a diagnostic dilemma, unless they have been given in large quantities prior to placement of the FHR monitor. If this occurs (Fig. 12–1) the reduction in variability can be profound. However, usually the drugs are given after an initial normal FHR tracing has been obtained, and the time course of change of variability, and its resolution after administration of the drug, allows one to logically relate the cause to the effect (Fig. 12–2).

A further effect of some narcotics has been described as the pseudosinusoidal pattern (see Fig. 9–24), which can generally be distinguished from the regular smooth true sinusoidal pattern. Once again, the relationship of

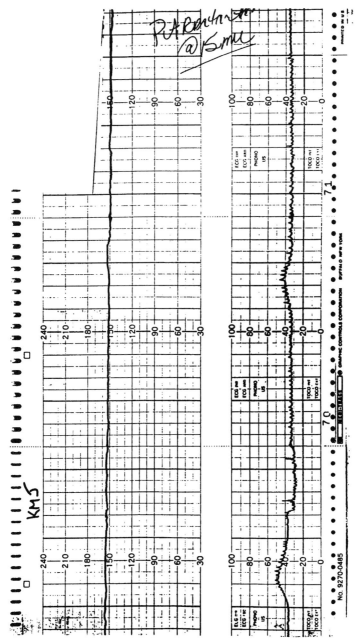

**FIGURE 12–1.** This near-term mother had received large doses of meperidine, 75 mg q2h, for unremitting pain from a renal stone, and labor was induced to allow definitive urologic treatment. The fetal blood pH was 7.3, confirming a drug-induced, nonasphyxial cause of absent FHR variability. The absence of periodic FHR changes also supports the nonasphyxial source of FHR variability reduction. The baby was born vaginally, and was normal. Fetal scalp electrode.

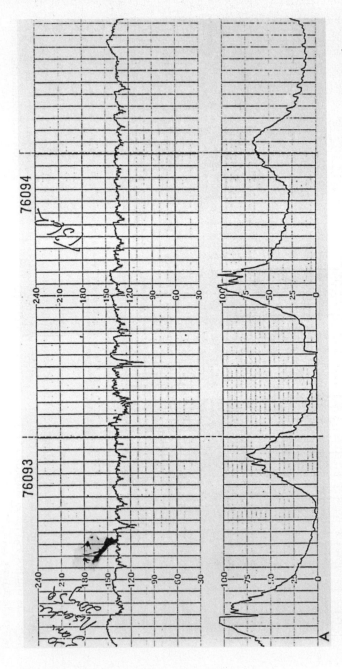

**FIGURE 12-2.** FHR before (A) and 15 minutes after (B) 20 mg of a narcotic, alphaprodine (Nisentil), was administered subcutaneously to the mother. Note the decrease in FHR variability after maternal absorption and presumed transplacental fetal uptake. The variability usually returns in approximately 45 minutes. The absence of decelerations or a bradycardia before the reduction in FHR variability confirms the nonasphyxial cause of the reduction.

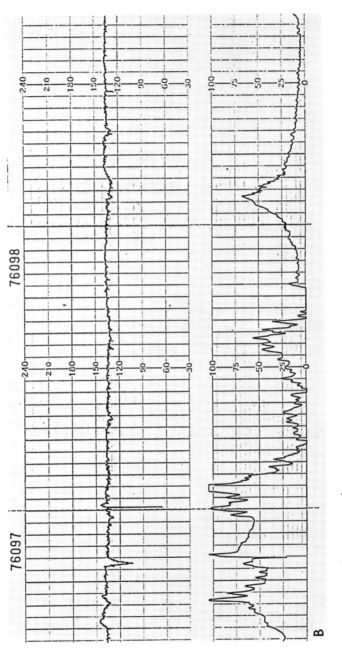

**FIGURE 12–2.** *Continued*

the time of administration of the drug to the onset and resolution of the pseudosinusoidal pattern is usually diagnostic.

The potential dilemma which may occur is during uncorrectable periodic changes when narcotics are given. If this results in a reduction in FHR variability it may be difficult to decide between asphyxial decompensation and drug effect. A number of factors minimize this dilemma. Firstly, narcotics often result in no change in FHR variability, and rarely result in abolition of variability, but more likely will cause transient reduction. One may be able to distinguish between asphyxial decompensation and drug effect by judging whether the depth of decelerations is sufficient to cause the reduction of variability, and the time course of alteration of variability. It should not be believed that narcotics are absolutely contraindicated in mothers with persistent periodic changes if pain relief is required. If a dilemma is presented, stimulation testing or (if available) fetal blood sampling can often resolve the question of asphyxial decompensation.

Parasympatholytic drugs, such as atropine or scopolamine, may cause a reduction in variability, or, if a total blocking dose reaches the fetus, may result in abolition of FHR variability (Fig. 12–3). Such drugs are usually given to the mother in relatively small doses, and in fact may cause no change in variability. However, in the early studies of FHR patterns a number of fetuses had direct administration of atropine, and profound effects on variability, and on vagally induced periodic patterns, were seen[1, 6, 7] (Fig. 12–4).

# D Congenital Abnormalities, Either Developmental or Acquired

There are numerous case reports in the literature regarding the association between an unremitting flat baseline and neurologic damage, and several relatively large series[8, 10, 11] showing the generally poor outlook for these babies. It should be stressed that the variability in most of these reports is not just reduced but virtually undetectable (Fig. 12–5). Although the exact etiology of the loss of variability is usually not known, it is assumed that such fetuses have suffered an asphyxial, ischemic, or toxic event of such severity that the cerebral cortex and/or other parts of the central nervous system are damaged to the extent that neurologic integrity of variability pathways is lost.

A number of principles with respect to these studies need to be considered.

1. The fact that many babies with neurologic damage have absent FHR variability does not necessarily mean that all babies with this pattern have neurologic damage. The subjects in some studies have been selected from medical litigation cases, where there is no suit unless there is damage, and similarly not often is a suit pressed unless there is an

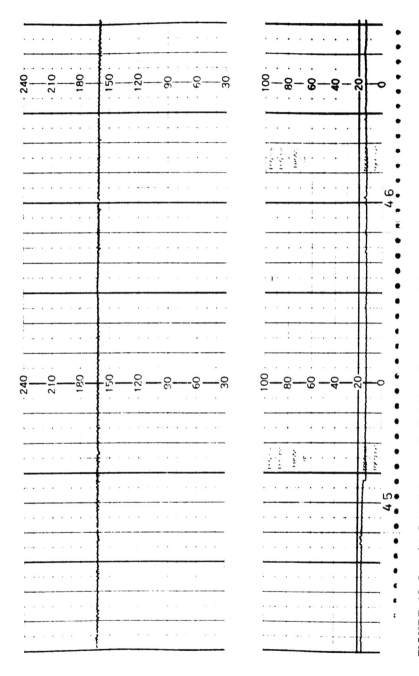

**FIGURE 12–3.** This flat FHR is a result of a 200-mg intraperitoneal dose of atropine in a 25-week fetus. The fetus had unexplained recurrent decelerations during an intraperitoneal fetal blood transfusion for erythroblastosis fetalis. The slight jitter mimicking short-term variability on the tracing probably represents Doppler ultrasound artifact.

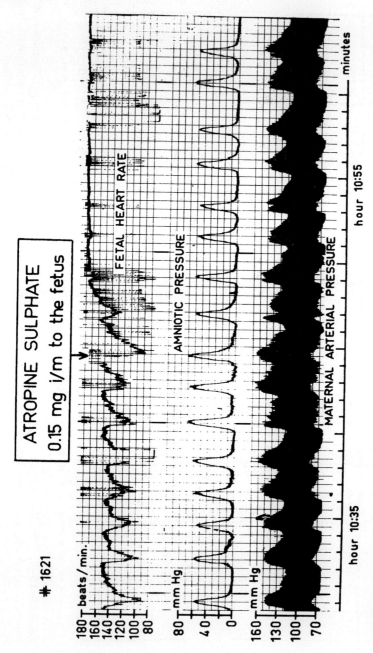

**FIGURE 12–4.** This fetus has variable decelerations and apparently normal FHR variability at 7 cm cervical dilation. The parasympatholytic drug atropine was administered, and several minutes later the decelerations and FHR variability were abolished, and a tachycardia developed. The tracing was obtained at 1 cm/min paper speed. (From Caldeyro-Barcia R, Mendez-Bauer C, Poseiro JJ, et al. Control of human fetal heart rate during labor. In Cessels DE, ed. The Heart and Circulation in the Newborn and Infant. Grune & Stratton, New York, 1966. Used by permission.)

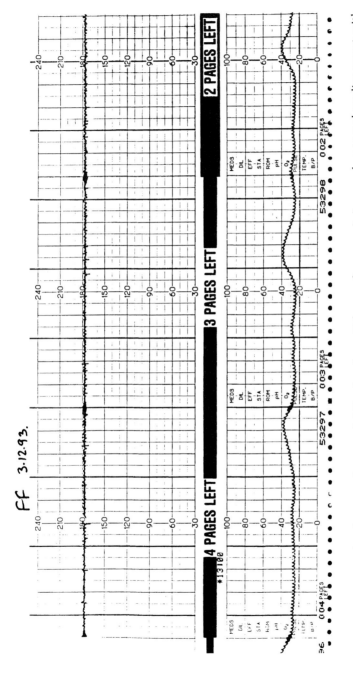

**FIGURE 12–5.** The absence of FHR variability in a fetus 12 hours after a semiwitnessed maternal cardiac arrest, with an FHR of 40 beats/min being recorded approximately 15 minutes after the arrest. The baby was born approximately 1 month later to the comatose mother, and had profound neurologic damage. FHR variability was never regained. Doppler ultrasound.

"abnormal" FHR tracing. So the FHR pattern and the damage are selected together, thus biasing the view that the flat trace always signifies damage.

2. The extreme case of absence of the higher centers in anencephaly results in a reduction in variability, sometimes to its absence.[3] There is evidence that the amount of variability remaining in anencephalics is related to the amount of midbrain tissue present.[12] This latter can vary quite widely in anencephalics. These observations have given rise to the view that the cerebral cortex is an important contributor to variability—maybe the most important—but some variability has its origin in some of the lower centers of the central nervous system.

3. It is possible to have profound neurologic or other impairment without any reduction in FHR variability. That is, the neuronal pathways of FHR variability may be intact, but there may be concomitant severe damage or malstructure in other parts of the central nervous system. Such neurologic pathology may be either developmental or acquired. Examples of developmental problems are disorders of neuronal migration, and chromosomal aneuploidy or deletions. Acquired neurologic deficits may be due to global ischemic/asphyxial events, or localized infarcts due to regional ischemia (strokes). Such defects are not always obvious on fetal sonographic imaging.

An unusual, though rarely difficult to diagnose condition, is seen in the fetus with complete heart block. Such fetuses lack FHR variability, as there is no transmission of atrial impulses across the atrioventricular node (see Fig. 7–10). In addition, they have an idioventricular rate of about 50 to 60 beats/min. In addition to lacking FHR variability, they should not have reflex periodic changes because of lack of a vagal connection to the ventricle.

## E   Severe Cerebral Asphyxia/Ischemia

The theory has been put forward, and not yet refuted, that some fetuses are so deeply asphyxiated that they have lost FHR variability, and no longer have the ability or mechanism to produce periodic FHR changes. Thus they have a flat heart rate within the normal range and death in utero would occur with a terminal bradycardia even in the presence of contractions. Such fetuses therefore act like the severely asphyxiated fetus in the antepartum period, where there are no decelerations because of the absence of contractions to trigger them. On the other hand, antepartum terminal patterns have been reported with a flat baseline and late decelerations, sometimes deep and prolonged, occurring with the rare intermittent prelabor contractions.[2, 4, 5, 13]

## F Sinusoidal Patterns

As noted in definitions of the components of the various FHR patterns (see Chapter 9), the sinusoidal pattern is a specific exclusion from FHR variability, despite the measurable amplitude of FHR fluctuation, usually with a frequency of 3 to 6/min (see Figs. 9–22 and 9–23).

The most common accompaniment to persistent sinusoidal patterns is fetal anemia, most often seen with severe erythroblastosis fetalis or fetal–maternal hemorrhage. Management of the sinusoidal pattern is described in Chapter 9.

 MANAGEMENT OF THE FETUS WITH AN INITIAL UNREMITTING FLAT BASELINE

Some guidelines to management have been given in the above categories, and a proposed schema from Nijuis and coworkers[8] is given in Table 12–1. However, there will still be some fetuses which present the clinician with a dilemma during labor (i.e., a flat unremitting baseline, with absence of periodic changes, no response to stimulation testing, and no known congenital anomalies). In such cases the only practical way to determine that the fetus is normoxic is by an intrapartum biophysical profile (although this has not been proven useful) or fetal blood sampling for acid-base measurement. If such ancillary testing is not possible or unavailable, or if the results are equivocal, then clinical judgment must be used in the management of the case, although most subspecialists would be reluctant to intervene operatively. It is valuable to obtain umbilical cord blood gases at the time of birth

**TABLE 12–1. Proposed Management of the Fetus Entering Labor With Unremitting Absent Fetal Heart Rate Variability**

| Differential Diagnosis | Action |
| --- | --- |
| Non-REM sleep state (state 1F) | Extend recording time<br>Exclude use of drugs |
| Anomalies | Ultrasound imaging<br>Behavioral observations (biophysical profile) |
| Hypoxia | Contraction stress test |
| Brain death | Fetal blood acid-base measurement |

Modified from Nijhuis JG, Crevels AJ, Van Dongen PWJ. Fetal brain death: The definition of a fetal heart rate pattern and its clinical consequences. Obstet Gynecol Surv 1990; 45:229–232.

to determine fetal acid base status, so that the subsequent medical review of the case can be facilitated.

# REFERENCES

1. Caldeyro-Barcia R, Mendez-Bauer C, Poseiro JJ, et al. Control of human fetal heart rate during labor. In Cassels DE, ed. The Heart and Circulation in the Newborn and Infant. Grune & Stratton, New York, 1966.

2. Cetrulo CL, Schifrin BS. Fetal heart rate patterns preceding death in utero. Obstet Gynecol 1976; 48:521–527.

3. deHaan J, van Bemmel JH, Stolte LAM, et al. Quantitative evaluation of fetal heart rate patterns II. The significance of fixed heart rate pattern during pregnancy and labor. Eur J Obstet Gynec 1971; 3:103–113.

4. Emmen L, Huisjes JJ, Aarnoudse JG, et al. Antepartum diagnosis of the "terminal" fetal state by cardiotocography. Br J Obstet Gynaecol 1975; 82:353–359.

5. Gaziano EP, Freeman DW. Analysis of heart rate patterns preceding fetal death. Obstet Gynecol 1977; 50:578–582.

6. Hon EH, Bradfield AH, Hess OW. The electronic evaluation of the fetal heart rate. V. The vagal factor in fetal bradycardia. Am J Obstet Gynecol 1961; 82:291–300.

7. Mendez-Bauer C, Poseiro JJ, Arellano-Hernandez G, et al. Effects of atropine on the heart rate of the human fetus during labor. Am J Obstet Gynecol 1963; 85:1033–1053.

8. Nijhuis JG, Crevels AJ, Van Dongen PWJ. Fetal brain death: The definition of a fetal heart rate pattern and its clinical consequences. Obstet Gynecol Survey 1990; 45:229–232.

9. Nijuis JG, Prechtl HFR, Martin CB Jr., Bots RSGM. Are there behavioural states in the human fetus? Early Hum Dev 1982; 6:177–195.

10. Phelan JP, Ahn MO. Perinatal observations in forty-eight neurologically impaired term infants. Am J Obstet Gynecol 1994; 171:424–431.

11. Schifrin BS, Hamilton-Rubinstein R, Shields JR. Fetal heart rate patterns and the timing of fetal injury. J Perinatol 1994; 14:174–181.

12. Terao T, Kawashima Y, Noto H, et al. Neurologic control of fetal heart rate in 20 cases of anencephalic fetuses. Am J Obstet Gynecol 1984; 149:201–208.

13. Tushuizen PB Th, Stoot JEGM, Ubachs JMH. Fetal heart rate monitoring of the dying fetus. Am J Obstet Gynecol 1974; 120:922–931.

# ■ *Chapter Thirteen*

# Second-Stage Patterns

There are many reasons for believing that management of fetal heart rate (FHR) patterns in the second stage should be different from that earlier in labor. Part of this is due to the proximity of delivery, and the possibility of a rapid operative vaginal delivery should the fetus show signs of asphyxial deterioration. In this chapter we will examine differences in the second stage, and offer some recommendations.

## I WHY MAY THE SECOND STAGE BE DIFFERENT?

### A Influence of Increases in Intraamniotic Pressure on Uterine Blood Flow

It is now well established that increases in intraamniotic pressure result in a decrease in uterine blood flow. This has been determined by direct measurements in various nonhuman species[3, 5, 6, 13] and inferentially from indirect measurements in the human.[2] There is, furthermore, evidence that the decrease in uterine blood flow is greater with higher increases in amniotic fluid pressure.

It is also known that fetal blood oxygen tension and content decrease with uterine contractions[8, 9] and that the reduction in fetal oxygen tension is related to the intensity of the contraction or with the degree of reduction of uterine blood flow (Fig. 13–1).

It might therefore be expected that in a fetus in which oxygenation is adequate at rest before labor, there will need to be a sufficient "reserve" of

**235**

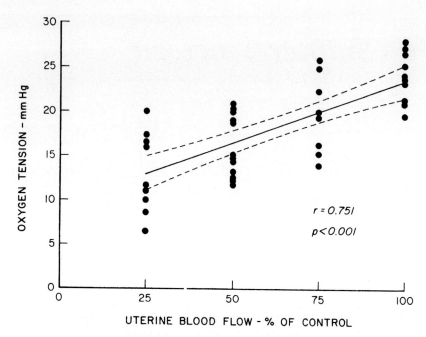

**FIGURE 13–1.** Relationship between the fetal umbilical arterial oxygen tension and percentage of baseline uterine blood flow in fetal sheep. (Modified from Yaffe H, Parer JT, Block BS, Llanos AJ. Cardiorespiratory responses to graded reductions of uterine blood flow in the sheep fetus. J Dev Physiol 1987; 9:325–336.)

oxygen delivery capacity to tolerate the transient reductions of oxygen delivery with contractions. Obviously, the vast majority of fetuses have this sufficient reserve, and do not have heart rate responses to contractions. However, essentially all fetuses develop a mild mixed respiratory and metabolic acidosis during labor, probably because of the cumulative effects of oxygen limitation in vasoconstricted vascular beds (see Chapter 6). However, in a fetus with compromised placental function (e.g., where there are placental infarctions due to hypertensive disease), there may be insufficient redundancy of uterine blood flow between contractions to avoid the development of a cumulative asphyxia.

Again, a fetus well oxygenated during the uterine contractions of the first-stage active phase of labor may be insufficiently oxygenated when intrauterine pressure exceeds 100 mmHg with pushing efforts in the second stage of labor (Fig. 13–2).

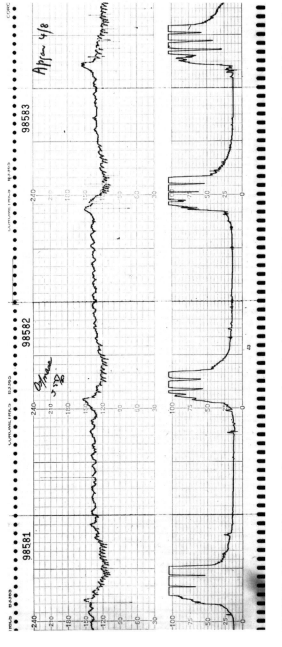

**FIGURE 13–2.** This normally grown term fetus had a normal FHR tracing up until the second stage of labor. Reflex late decelerations probably began then as a result of further decreases in uterine blood flow and peripheral fetal oxygen tension with the high intraamniotic pressure during pushing. A normal fetus was delivered.

# B  Influence of Uterine Contractions on Umbilical Blood Flow

A commonly stated view is that variable decelerations are due to compression of the umbilical cord, which because of the increased intraamniotic pressure during contractions, is generally considered to be more likely to occur during these periods. There is some support for this in cases of oligohydramnios, either primary or after rupture of membranes, as the variable decelerations can sometimes be abolished by infusion of saline into the amniotic cavity.[10, 11] It is, however, difficult to discern why there should be cord compression inside the amniotic cavity of the fetus with a normal amount of amniotic fluid, as the pressure should be transmitted equally throughout the whole of the vascular system of the fetus. Against this, however, there is some evidence of alteration in thoracic dimensions in fetal sheep during spontaneous prelabor uterine contractions.[7]

Compression of the umbilical cord will cause a decrease in umbilical blood flow. The lower hydrostatic pressure in the umbilical vein will cause it to be compressed more than the umbilical artery, so venous return to the fetus is first reduced. This may cause certain FHR responses, and there is evidence in fetal goat that the initial response is a tachycardia.[14] With more severe compression there is constriction of the umbilical artery, so circulation of oxygen-poor blood from the fetus to the placenta is reduced. The mechanism causing heart rate responses due to this could be an increase in afterload, causing an increased arterial blood pressure, and reduction in FHR by the baroreflex. The resulting cyanosis due to reduced placental circulation may also cause a bradycardia due to vagal activity by the chemoreflex. Under conditions of severe and prolonged umbilical cord compression there may also be bradycardia due to myocardial hypoxia.

Variable decelerations are more common during the second stage of labor than earlier, and there is increasing evidence that it is not cord compression at this time, but rather vagal reflexes due to dural stimulation as the head is squeezed while being compressed against the bony pelvis or resistant vaginal tissues during voluntary pushing efforts (Fig. 13–3). If this is indeed the mechanism then it may not be caused by hypoxia, but it could conceivably be a cause of fetal hypoxia due to decreased fetal cardiac output and umbilical blood flow (see Chapter 9).

Severe variable decelerations are not infrequently seen with traction on forceps or the vacuum extractor, presumably due to the same mechanism of dural stimulation (Fig. 13–4).

An earlier view based on studies in fetal sheep suggested that fetal cardiac output was dependent on heart rate, with a poor capacity to increase stroke volume during decreases in heart rate.[12] It now seems that this is not universally true, as the sheep fetus can increase its stroke volume under conditions of

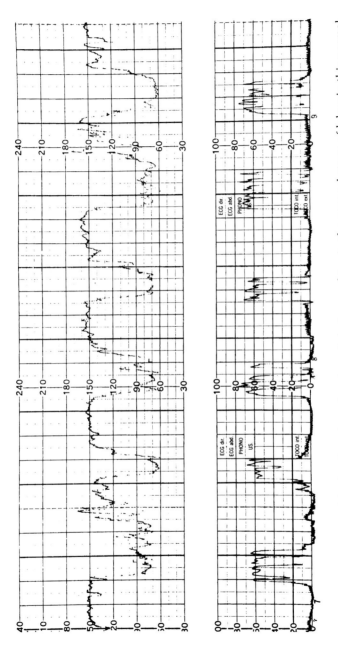

**FIGURE 13–3.**  Variable decelerations developed during pushing in the second stage of labor in this normal, term fetus. The decelerations represent vagal activity most likely as a result of dural stimulation due to head compression. Fetal heart rate variability is maintained and a normal fetus resulted.

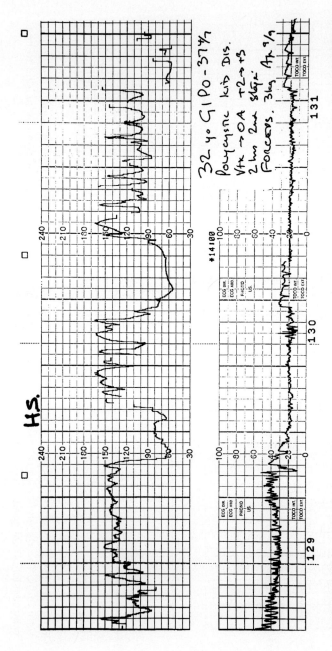

**FIGURE 13–4.** Three severe variable decelerations developed in this otherwise essentially normal FHR tracing during traction with forceps. It is presumed that the decelerations were due to vagal stimulation from head compression. The baby was delivered during the final deceleration, and was normal.

hypoxic bradycardia[4] and pacing.[1] However, in the fetus as in the adult, when heart rate is very low the Frank–Starling mechanism can no longer compensate and cardiac output and umbilical blood flow fall to unacceptable levels (see Chapter 4). Clinical experience suggests that this may not occur until the FHR falls to values below 60 beats/min (see Chapters 9 and 11).

## II MANAGEMENT RECOMMENDATIONS FOR THE SECOND STAGE OF LABOR

There are two features which set the second stage apart with respect to management. First, the appearance of decelerations and bradycardias is far more common in the second stage than earlier in labor. Second, expeditious and relatively safe vaginal delivery is generally readily accomplished operatively or with an episiotomy in the second stage.

Intervention in the second stage in the presence of late or severe variable decelerations with good FHR variability can almost always await the advancement of the vertex to a low station. One can also frequently adhere to maternal desires with respect to episiotomy or an operative delivery.

Prolonged bradycardias are not infrequent preceding and during expulsion of the fetal head. As noted above, there is no urgent reason to intervene provided the baseline FHR is above 60 beats/min and FHR variability is maintained (Fig. 13–5). On occasion one will hear of cases where an operative delivery is carried out for "fetal distress" for such a pattern. This should preferably be referred to as an optional form of management (Fig. 13–6). However, the conservative approach to second-stage patterns should not necessarily lull one into a false sense of complacency regarding the frequently bizarre patterns which can be seen in the second stage. Patterns can evolve quite rapidly into those signifying fetal asphyxia, so preparation for delivery must be such that it can be accomplished rapidly should the situation so warrant (see Fig. 11–2).

In summary, the attendants during labor should be aware of the additional stresses placed on the fetal oxygen supply line during the second stage, as reflected by changes in the FHR pattern. This awareness should, however, be tempered by the knowledge that the majority of fetuses tolerate these stresses quite well, and potentially hazardous intervention is rarely necessary. However, because of the possibility, albeit uncommon, of rapid decompensation, facilities for rapid intervention should be available.

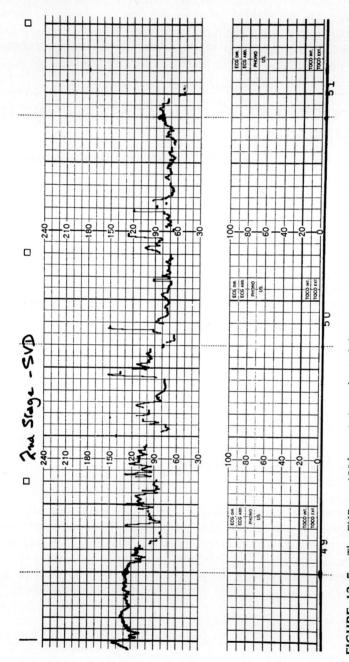

**FIGURE 13–5.** The FHR was 130 beats/min and variability normal in this term fetus until the final 7 minutes before delivery, when a bradycardia with normal FHR variability occurred. The mother's desire for a spontaneous delivery was adhered to, and a normal baby was the result.

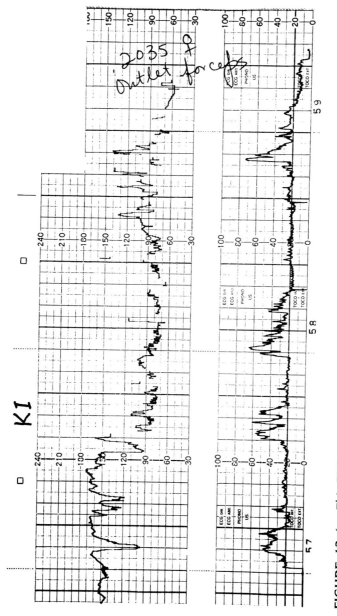

**FIGURE 13–6.** This FHR tracing was normal until the head was on the pelvic floor, and a deceleration of approximately 70 to 100 beats/min with good variability occurred for approximately 6 minutes. Delivery was accomplished by outlet forceps. This is an acceptable but not mandatory mode of delivery in such cases. A 2840-g baby with Apgar scores of 6 (1 minute) and 9 (5 minutes) was the result.

# REFERENCES

1. Anderson PAW, Glick KL, Killam AP, Mainwaring RD. The effect of heart rate on *in utero* left ventricular output in the fetal sheep. J Physiol 1986; 372:557–573.

2. Brotanek V, Hendricks CM, Yoshida T. Changes in uterine blood flow during contractions. Am J Obstet Gynecol 1969; 103:1108–1111.

3. Cabalum T, Nathanielsz PW. The effect of episodes of tonic myometrial activity on common uterine artery blood flow in the pregnant sheep at 110 to 135 days gestation. J Physiol 1981; 320:104P.

4. Cohn HE, Sacks EJ, Heymann MA, Rudolph AM. Cardiovascular response to hypoxemia and acidemia in fetal lambs. Am J Obstet Gynecol 1974; 120:817–824.

5. Greiss FC Jr. Effect of labor on uterine blood flow. Observations on gravid ewes. Am J Obstet Gynecol 1965; 93:917.

6. Harbert GM Jr. Uterine contractions. Clin Obstet Gynecol 1982; 25:177–187.

7. Harding R, Poore ER. The effects of myometrial activity on fetal thoracic dimensions and uterine blood flow during late gestation in the sheep. Biol Neonate 1984; 45:244–252.

8. Jansen CAM, Krane EJ, Thomas AL, et al. Continuous variability of fetal $pO_2$ in the chronically catheterized fetal sheep. Am J Obstet Gynecol 1979; 134:776–784.

9. Llanos AJ, Court DJ, Block BS, et al. Fetal cardiorespiratory changes during spontaneous prelabor uterine contractions in sheep. Am J Obstet Gynecol 1986; 155:893–897.

10. Miyazaki FS, Nevarez F. Saline amnioinfusion for relief of repetitive variable decelerations: A prospective randomized study. Am J Obstet Gynecol 1985; 153:301–306.

11. Nageotte MP, Freeman RK, Garite TJ, Dorchchester W. Prophylactic intrapartum amnioinfusion in patients with preterm premature rupture of membranes. Am J Obstet Gynecol 1985; 153:557–565.

12. Rudolph AM, Heymann MA. Cardiac output in the fetal lamb: The effects of spontaneous and induced changes of heart rate on right and left ventricular output. Am J Obstet Gynecol 1976; 124:183–191.

13. Sunderji SG, El Badry A, Poore ER, et al. The effect of myometrial contractures on uterine blood flow in the pregnant sheep at 114 to 140 days gestation measured by the 4-aminoantipyrine equilibrium diffusion technique. Am J Obstet Gynecol 1984; 149:408–418.

14. Towell ME, Salvador HS. Compression of the umbilical cord: An experimental model in the fetal goat. In Crosignani PG, Pardi G, eds. Fetal Evaluation during Pregnancy and Labor. Academic Press, New York, 1971, p. 143.

# ■ *Chapter Fourteen*

# Labor Management

Two advances in recent decades have aided the rational management of labor: (1) the cervical dilatation–fetal descent versus time curve largely developed by Friedman,[7–9] and (2) the intrapartum monitor, which allows one to quantitate uterine activity (see Chapter 7).

Labor is a dynamic process by which regular uterine activity propels the fetus through the lower uterine segment, the bony pelvis, the cervix, and the vagina in a fashion that generally is predictable. These anatomic structures provide a resistance to the passage of the fetus, and the uterine contractions provide the force to overcome the resistance.

The factors affecting blood flow have been discussed previously (see Chapter 3), namely:

$$\text{Blood flow} = \frac{\text{Arteriovenous blood pressure difference}}{\text{Vascular resistance}}$$

This formula is directly applicable to the "flow" of the fetus from the uterus to the outside world (Fig. 14–1):

$$\text{Rate of passage of fetus} = \frac{\text{Intraamniotic pressure} - \text{Atmospheric pressure}}{\text{Resistance of pelvic tissues}}$$

The uterine activity can be quantitated by taking continuous measurements of intrauterine pressure. The resistance cannot be measured accurately, even by x-ray pelvimetry. Excessive resistance can, however, be surmized from inadequate progress (i.e., inadequate dilatation or fetal descent) in the face of adequate uterine activity.

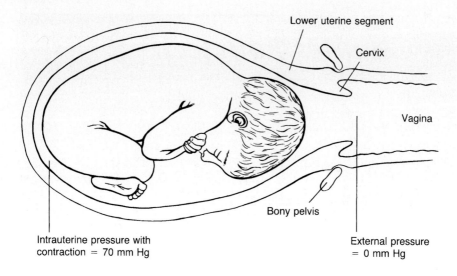

Lower uterine segment

Cervix

Vagina

Bony pelvis

Intrauterine pressure with
contraction = 70 mm Hg

External pressure
= 0 mm Hg

$$\text{Rate of Passage} = \frac{\text{Pressure difference}}{\text{Resistance of pelvic tissues}}$$

**FIGURE 14–1.** A schematic depiction of the factors involved in the speed of passage of the fetus during birth.

# I    UTERINE ACTIVITY

Uterine activity is measured by the second channel of the fetal monitor (see Chapter 7). The external tokodynamometer can conveniently record uterine contraction frequency and duration but is unable to quantify intensity in normal clinical practice. The internal mode—the catheter and the strain-gauge transducer—can monitor contraction frequency, duration, and intensity, and another potentially important quality, uterine tonus.

In active labor, contractions generally occur every 2 to 3 minutes. They last 60 seconds or more and have an intensity of 50 to 80 mmHg. The baseline tonus (i.e., the pressure of the amniotic fluid between uterine contractions) is generally 10 to 15 mmHg. There are a number of methods of combining the contraction frequency and the intensity in order to quantify uterine activity, but the simplest and most widespread technique is to use the Montevideo unit, developed by one of the pioneers of monitoring, Roberto Caldeyro-Barcia of Montevideo, Uruguay.

Montevideo units (MU) are the product of the number of uterine contractions in 10 minutes multiplied by the mean intensity of the contraction in millimeters of mercury. Clinically, the value is obtained roughly by adding together the peak intensities of each contraction in a 10-minute period (Fig. 14–2).

In active-phase spontaneous labor, uterine activity usually does not exceed 280 MU (i.e., contractions approximately 3 minutes apart and 90 mmHg in intensity).[4] Hence, if progress is inadequate (as determined by progressive cervical dilatation), one is justified in augmenting it with oxytocin if uterine activity is below this level. It generally is thought (although the opinion is based on evidence that is rather poor) that exceeding this level of activity may result in rupture of the uterus or fetal damage. Originally, Caldeyro-Barcia defined the MU by subtracting the tonus from the peak values for each contraction. It is operationally simpler to use the combined values for each peak, and aim for progressive cervical dilatation or 280 MU with oxytocin augmentation, whichever comes first.

The dosage of oxytocin used to initiate or augment labor is currently under much scrutiny, and will not be covered in this book. Opinions range from low-dose, slow-increase[13] to aggressive, early use of relatively large doses of oxytocin.[12]

Clinically, one can determine frequency by palpation, but there is little doubt that use of the monitor (either the tokodynamometer or the intrauterine catheter) is more accurate and convenient. Another advantage is that this equipment leaves a permanent record. Intensity also can be determined by palpation and, with experience, it probably can be ascertained fairly accurately. Intensity by palpation generally is judged on a scale of 1+ to 4+. Again, however, the catheter technique is more convenient, and risks with the use of the device appear to be minimal (see Chapter 15).

## II  CERVICAL DILATATION AND DESCENT OF THE FETUS

Cervical dilatation, estimated digitally in centimeters, can be graphed against time to give certain patterns of progress.[7–9] In addition, when the station of the presenting part is determined, a second pattern can be graphed on the same curve (Fig. 14–3). These patterns are conveniently divided into certain phases and stages, and various expected durations and their outside limits for each period have been determined both for nulliparas and for multiparas.[7–9, 11]

The onset of labor is defined as the beginning of regular, frequent (every 5 minutes), intense contractions that persist until delivery. Admittedly, the

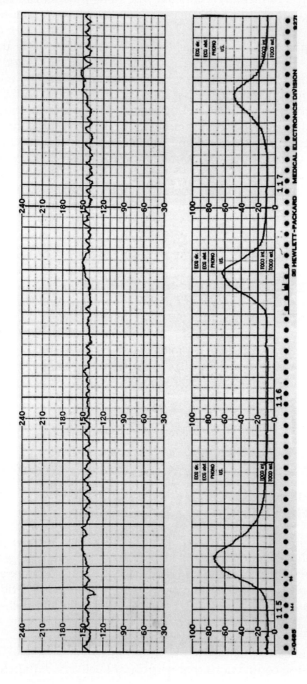

**FIGURE 14–2.** The calculation of Montevideo units (MU). In this 10-minute period, there are three uterine contractions of 73, 63, and 50 mmHg peak intensity, so there are 186 MU.

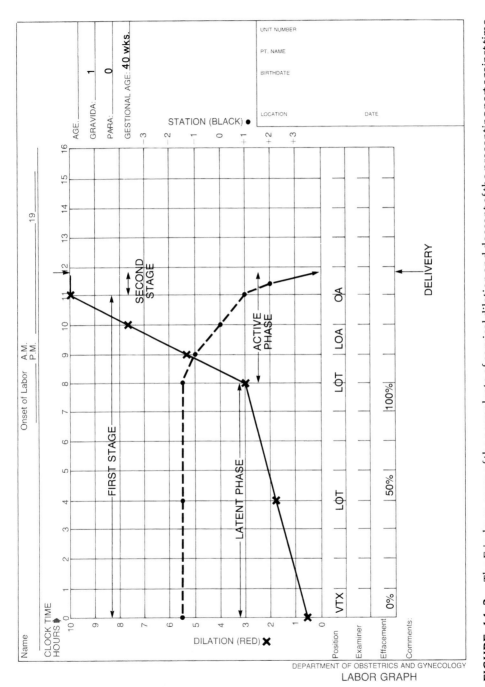

**FIGURE 14-3.** The Friedman curve of the normal rate of cervical dilation and descent of the presenting part against time. Also shown are the stages and phases of labor.

time of onset sometimes is difficult to determine, because each pregnant mother's sensation of "intensity" varies.

There are two stages of labor. The first stage begins with the onset of labor and ends with complete cervical dilatation. The first stage consists of two phases, latent and active (Fig. 14–3).

The latent phase commences with the onset of labor and ends at the beginning of rapid dilatation (i.e., at the break in the cervical dilatation curve). It should be noted that strictly speaking one can determine the end of the latent phase only after the active phase has begun. An important event in the latent phase is progressive cervical effacement, which is considered an advancement during this period, particularly in nulliparas.

The active phase consists of the time of rapid cervical dilatation and ends with delivery of the baby, so the active phase encompasses part of the first stage and all of the second stage.

The second stage of labor begins with complete dilatation and ends with delivery of the baby.

Mean time intervals of each of these subdivisions have been measured in nulliparous and multiparous patients (Table 14–1). These figures come as a surprise to many trainees in obstetrics, who generally expect much longer mean values. It must be remembered, however, that the range of duration is very large, and that generally those patients who have prolonged labor are more obvious and receive special recognition because of the need for extra caution or intervention.

---

# III   ABNORMALITIES OF LABOR

Only five abnormalities can occur during the progress of labor: (1) prolonged latent phase, (2) protracted or slow slope active phase, (3) active phase arrest, (4) prolonged second stage, and (5) failure of fetal descent. Each of these abnormalities is readily recognized graphically. Various time criteria are used to define these abnormalities, and these numbers generally represent values that are conveniently rounded off at approximately the mean plus 2 standard deviations. In addition, for simplicity, some distinctions between values for nulliparas and values for multiparas have been omitted. Such mathematical conveniences are of no particular significance from the patient's point of view, since the definitions are primarily for communication and statistical classification and do not represent a call for any immediate or drastic action. These abnormalities and their possible causes and treatments will be discussed in the following sections. It should be noted that the simplified statements made in the tables are discussed and qualified in the following text.

TABLE 14–1.  **Mean Time Intervals During Labor**

|  | Primipara | Multipara |
|---|---|---|
| **First stage** | | |
| Latent phase | 7 hr | 4 hr |
| Active phase | 4 hr | 2 hr |
| **Second stage** | 50 min | 20 min |

Modified from Ledger WJ. Monitoring of labor by graphs. Obstet Gynecol 1969; 34:174–187.

# A  Prolonged Latent Phase

A *prolonged latent phase of labor* is defined as a latent phase of greater that 12 hours in multiparas, and 18 hours in nulliparas:

| Possible Causes | Possible Treatments |
|---|---|
| **Unfavorable cervix** | Administer narcotics and prescribe rest |
| | Augment with oxytocin |
| | Apply prostaglandin to cervix |
| **Abnormal uterine activity** | |
| Primary | Administer narcotics, prescribe rest, or give oxytocin |
| Secondary | |
| Oversedation | Correct secondary causes; |
| Anesthesia | administer oxytocin |
| Dehydration | |

It should be noted that fetopelvic disproportion is not a cause of a prolonged latent phase. The major difficulty with this abnormality occurs if the membranes are ruptured in the presence of an unfavorable cervix, because the longer the period of rupture, after a certain threshold interval, the greater the risk of infection. Hence, if no progress is made in effacement (or dilatation) after 12 or 18 hours of 280 MU there arises the possibility of a failed augmentation. Prostaglandin applied to the cervix may be used to improve the Bishop's score.

There are the other cases where induction is desired, either for maternal or fetal indications, and the patient must be "given" a latent phase, either with cervical prostaglandin treatment or oxytocin. Without acute maternal or fetal jeopardy, or ruptured membranes, there is no particular time limit which must be applied to determine a failed induction.

Most of those patients who have prolonged latent phases will have unfavorable cervices (i.e., a low Bishop's score; Table 14–2), generally 0 to 3.[3] A patient with a Bishop's score greater than 9 will almost invariably enter

## TABLE 14–2. Bishop's Score

| Factor | Assigned Value | | | |
|---|---|---|---|---|
| | **0** | **1** | **2** | **3** |
| Cervical dilatation (cm) | Closed | 1–2 | 3–4 | 5 or more |
| Cervical effacement (%) | 0–25 | 25–50 | 50–75 | 75 or more |
| Fetal station | −3 | −2 | −1,0 | +1 or lower |
| Cervical consistency | Firm | Moderate | Soft | |
| Cervical position | Posterior | Midposition | Anterior | |

Modified from Bishop EH. Pelvic scoring for elective induction. Obstet Gyencol 1964; 24:266–268.

active labor within an hour or so after amniotomy. Patients with intermediate scores may need oxytocin in addition to amniotomy for successful induction.

## B Protracted Active Phase

A *protracted* or *slow-slope* active phase (Fig. 14–4) is defined as cervical dilatation of less than 1 cm/hr. There are slight differences for nullipares and multipares, but for descriptive and statistical purposes it is easier to use the simpler 1 cm/hr rate.

| Possible Causes | Possible Treatments |
|---|---|
| **Abnormal uterine activity** | |
| Primary | Administer oxytocin |
| Secondary | |
| Oversedation | Correct secondary causes; administer |
| Anesthesia | oxytocin if needed |
| Dehydration | |
| Fetopelvic disproportion | Perform cesarean section if diagnosis is firm, dilatation is persistently less than 1 cm/2 hrs, and/or 280 MU cannot be attained despite oxytocin |
| **Fetopelvic disproportion** | |
| Large fetus | Perform cesarean section if diagnosis is |
| Small pelvis (bony and | firm and dilatation is persistently less |
| soft tissue) | than 1 cm/2 hrs with oxytocin and adequate uterine stimulation (i.e., 280 MU) |
| Abnormal position | |

Sometimes, stimulation with oxytocin fails to produce the desired 280 MU despite doses of 30 mU/min or more. It appears that in some cases of fetopelvic disproportion, the uterus is resistant to stimulation and is prevented from

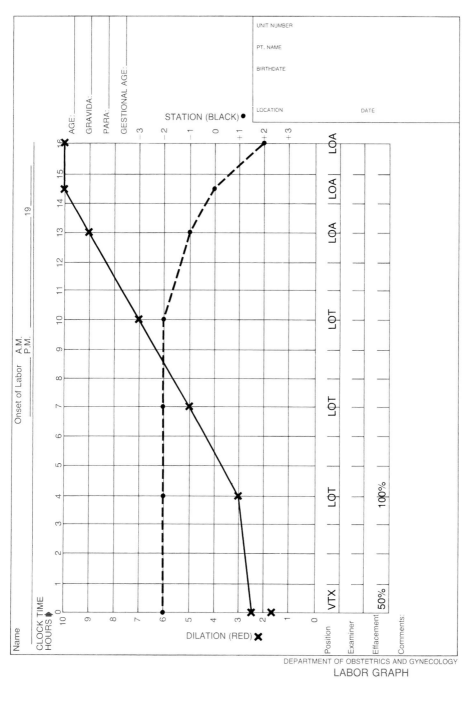

**FIGURE 14–4.** An abnormality of labor: the protracted or slow-slope active phase.

attaining its optimal level of activity. The mechanism by which this phenomenon occurs is unknown.

Determining fetopelvic disproportion in cases of this abnormality is the most difficult aspect of management. In a very small number of parturients, usually growing teenagers, the pelvis is obviously small on clinical examination. Often, these women are of small stature (less than 5 feet tall) and have a small shoe size, signifying overall decreased bone size and capacity. There is no good method of determining borderline disproportion. The clinical definition of *borderline disproportion* is notoriously inaccurate, and spontaneous vaginal delivery is seen in over 20 percent of mothers with "absolute disproportion" determined by x-ray pelvimetry.[6] In addition, inaccuracies occur in the converse situation (i.e., disproportion sometimes is seen even with an adequate bony pelvis, because soft tissue dystocia, particularly in obese patients, cannot adequately be taken into account on x-ray imaging).

There is, however, a dynamic definition of fetopelvic disproportion, that is, arrested dilatation despite adequate uterine activity for two or more hours (see the next section). This concept is difficult to apply in the slow-slope active-phase abnormality, because there is some progress, albeit minimal, in dilatation. The compromise reached is that if disproportion can be diagnosed clinically and progress is persistently less than 1 cm/2 hrs, cesarean section may be performed.

## C  Active-Phase Arrest

An *active-phase arrest* (Fig. 14–5) is defined as no dilatation in the active phase for 2 hours.

| Possible Causes | Possible Treatments |
| --- | --- |
| **Abnormal uterine activity** | |
| Primary | Administer oxytocin |
| Secondary | |
| Oversedation | Correct secondary causes; administer |
| Anesthesia | oxytocin if needed |
| Dehydration | |
| **Fetopelvic disproportion** | |
| Large fetus | Perform cesarean section if arrest per- |
| Small pelvis (bony and soft tissue) | sists for 2 to 3 hours with 280 MU |
| Abnormal position | |

Active-phase arrest is the easiest labor abnormality to manage and, as can be seen, it depends heavily on intraamniotic pressure measurements for its rapid diagnosis. This is actually the "dynamic" determination of fetopelvic disproportion and is not subject to the errors of determining "pelvic capacity" by clinical means or by x-ray studies.

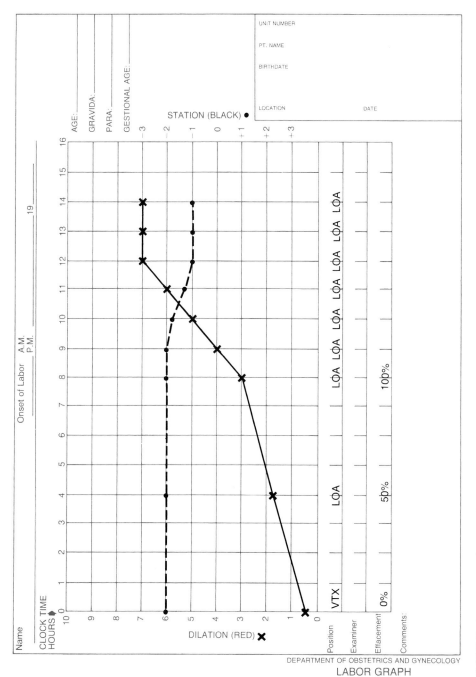

**FIGURE 14–5.**    An abnormality of labor: the active-phase arrest.

Active-phase arrest at the lower degrees of dilatation (e.g., 4 cm) can be difficult to diagnose, because it is difficult to know whether the patient is still in the latent phase. This phase can last several hours beyond 4 cm dilatation, or complete cervical effacement; hence, one should be reluctant to diagnose an arrest at this stage for three or more hours.

## D  Prolonged Second Stage

A *prolonged second stage* (Fig. 14–6) was in the past defined as a second stage lasting greater than two hours. It is closely related etiologically and therapeutically to the final disorder, failure of descent. Recent work has redefined these values, depending on the parity of the mother, and whether or not conduction anesthesia is used. The limits of "normal" are shown in Table 14–3, derived from the work of Kilpatrick and Laros,[10] and guidelines of the American College of Obstetricians and Gynecologists.[2] Nulliparous patients are at the 95th centile of the second stage in 2 hours without regional anesthesia, and in 3 hours with regional anesthesia. Parous patients are at the 95th centile if the second stage is 1 hour without regional anesthesia, and 2 hours with regional anesthesia.

## E  Failure of Descent

*Failure of descent* (Fig. 14–6) is defined as failure of the presenting part of the fetus to deliver after 1 to 3 hours in the second stage, depending on the factors outlined in Table 14–3.

The last two disorders will be discussed together.

| Possible Causes | Possible Treatments |
|---|---|
| **Abnormal uterine activity** | |
| Primary | Administer oxytocin |
| Secondary | |
| Oversedation | Correct secondary causes |
| Anesthesia | Administer oxytocin |
| Dehydration | Encourage voluntary effort |
| Inadequate voluntary | Operative vaginal delivery |
| effort | Wait |
| | See below |
| **Fetopelvic disproportion** | |
| Large fetus | Perform cesarean section if uterine activity and |
| Small pelvis (bony and soft | pushing have been adequate and diagnosis of |
| tissue) | fetopelvic disproportion is firm, or the vertex is |
| Abnormal position | at high station |
| | Trial of operative vaginal delivery (vacuum extractor or forceps) if diagnosis is uncertain; perform cesarean section if the trial fails |

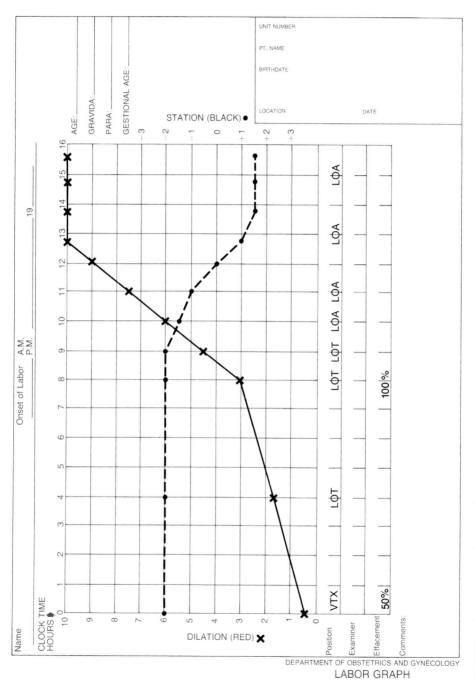

**FIGURE 14–6.** Two abnormalities of labor: the prolonged second stage and failure of descent.

**TABLE 14–3.   Lengths of First and Second Stages of Labor in Term Patients, With Singleton, Vertex Pregnancies, Delivering Vaginally Without Oxytocin for Induction or Augmentation**

| | No Conduction Anesthesia | | Conduction Anesthesia | |
|---|---|---|---|---|
| | *First Stage* (hr) | *Second Stage* (min) | *First Stage* (hr) | *Second Stage* (min) |
| **Nulliparous** | | | | |
| Mean ± SD | 8 ± 4 | 54 ± 39 | 10 ± 4 | 79 ± 53 |
| 95th centile | 17 | 132 | 19 | 185 |
| **Parous** | | | | |
| Mean ± SD | 6 ± 3 | 19 ± 21 | 7 ± 4 | 45 ± 43 |
| 95th centile | 13 | 61 | 15 | 131 |

Modified from Kilpatrick SJ, Laros RK Jr. Characteristics of normal labor. Obstet Gynecol 1989; 74:85–87.

The American College of Obstetricians and Gynecologists[1, 2] has redefined the descriptors for mid, low, and outlet forceps (Table 14–4).

These criteria and courses of action are meant to be guidelines only, and one must bear in mind the potentially traumatic results of difficult operative deliveries, particularly to the fetus. The judgment and skill required for such deliveries mandate the presence of a skilled member of the staff.

Continuous fetal heart rate (FHR) monitoring is recommended during the above labor abnormalities. There is no sound evidence that awaiting clarification of diagnosis does any traumatic damage to the fetus, even in the face of fetopelvic disproportion, provided reasonable time restrictions are observed and fetal asphyxia is excluded by continued FHR monitoring. The older idea that the second stage should be terminated at 2 hours to prevent fetal morbidity is no longer accepted since the demonstration that if asphyxia is ruled out there is no increase in adverse fetal outcome with a reasonable prolongation of the second stage.[5]

Reasons for prolonging the second stage beyond the statistical limits include

1. A strong desire for the mother to achieve a noninstrumented delivery.
2. Inability to push due to excessive sensory loss following a dense regional anesthesia.
3. Awaiting further descent and possibly head moulding to achieve a safer vaginal delivery.

Reasons for terminating the second stage include such factors as:

**1.** Maternal exhaustion.

**2.** Maternal medical conditions which precludes Valsalva maneuver.

**3.** Presumed or actual fetal asphyxia.

# IV SUMMARY

Labor difficulties can be recognized readily by graphic display of cervical dilatation and fetal descent against time. The causes of these abnormalities generally are inadequate uterine activity and excessive resistance of the lower pelvic tissues to passage of the fetus. The adequacy of uterine contractions can be reasonably well measured clinically and measured accurately and conveniently by the intrauterine catheter and the strain-gauge transducer of the fetal monitor. Uterine activity can be enhanced with oxytocin when appropriate, and fetopelvic disproportion can be diagnosed by exclusion. The concomitant use of continuous FHR monitoring during such diagnostic maneuvers is recommended in order to rule out the development of fetal asphyxia.

**TABLE 14–4. Criteria of Forceps Deliveries According to Station and Rotation**

| Types of Procedure | Criteria |
| --- | --- |
| Outlet forceps | Scalp is visible at the introitus without separating labia |
| | Fetal skull has reached pelvic floor |
| | Sagittal suture is in anteroposterior diameter or right or left occiput anterior or posterior position |
| | Fetal head is at or on perineum |
| | Rotation does not exceed 45 degrees |
| Low forceps | Leading point of fetal skull is at station +2 cm or more and not on the pelvic floor |
| | Rotation 45 degrees or less (left or right occiput anterior to occiput anterior, or left or right occiput posterior to occiput posterior) |
| | Rotation greater than 45 degrees |
| Midforceps | Station above +2 cm but head engaged |
| High | Not included in classification |

From ACOG Technical Bulletin No. 196. Operative vaginal delivery, Washington, DC, © ACOG August 1994.

# REFERENCES

1. American College of Obstetricians and Gynecologists. Obstetric forceps. ACOG Committee Opinions No. 59, 1988.

2. American College of Obstetricians and Gynecologists. Operative vaginal delivery. ACOG Technical Bulletins No. 196, 1994.

3. Bishop EH. Pelvic scoring for elective induction. Obstet Gynecol 1964; 24:266–268.

4. Caldeyro-Barcia R, Poseiro JJ. Oxytocin and contractility of the pregnant human uterus. Ann NY Acad Sci 1959; 72:813–830.

5. Cohen WR. Influence of the duration of second stage labor on perinatal outcome and puerperal morbidity. Obstet Gynecol 1977; 49:266–269.

6. Fine EA, Bracken M, Berkowitz RL. An evaluation of the usefulness of x-ray pelvimetry: Comparison of the Thoms and modified Ball methods with manual pelvimetry. Am J Obstet Gynecol 1980; 137:15–20.

7. Friedman EA. Primigravid labor. A graphicostatistical analysis. Obstet Gynecol 1955; 6:567–589.

8. Friedman EA. Labor in multiparas: A graphicostatistical analysis. Obstet Gynecol 1956; 8:691–703.

9. Friedman EA. Patterns of labor as indicators of risk. Clin Obstet Gynaecol 1973; 16:172–183.

10. Kilpatrick SJ, Laros RK Jr. Characteristics of normal labor. Obstet Gynecol 1989; 74:85–87.

11. Ledger WJ. Monitoring of labor by graphs. Obstet Gynecol 1969; 34:174–181.

12. O'Driscoll K, Foley M, MacDonald D. Active management of labour as an alternative to cesarean section for dystocia. Obstet Gynecol 1984; 63:485–490.

13. Seitchik J, Amico JA, Castillo M. Oxytocin augmentation of dysfunctional labor. V. An alternative oxytocin regimen. Am J Obstet Gynecol 1985; 151:757–761.

# Part Six

# OTHER ASPECTS OF MONITORING

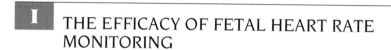

# ■ *Chapter Fifteen*

# Efficacy, Risks, and Recommendations for Usage

## I   THE EFFICACY OF FETAL HEART RATE MONITORING

### A  The Randomized Controlled Trials

The controlled trials of electronic fetal heart rate (FHR) monitoring have until recently shown little or no beneficial effect when compared with conventional management. This is not only puzzling but of great concern to many clinicians who believe electronic FHR monitoring is effective because of numerous clinical observations and the physiologic basis of FHR patterns. Many obstetricians can show cases in which the use of electronic FHR monitoring undoubtedly led to early intervention and lessening of continued intrapartum asphyxia. Nonetheless, for several reasons the trials have not consistently shown a beneficial effect and in fact have shown the detrimental effect of increased cesarean section rates in the monitored group.[15]

One reason for this lack of consistent benefit is that, in earlier trials particularly, patient numbers were inadequate to show a difference in mortality rates when the intrinsic rate is so low. Second, criteria used for diagnosis of fetal asphyxia were generally dated and unsophisticated, bearing little relationship to modern criteria. In particular, there had been little or no recognition of the importance of FHR variability in the determination of fetal status. The largest and most recent trial contains no description whatsoever of the FHR indices used to determine "abnormalities of fetal heart rate."[8] A further effect of unsophisticated FHR interpretation is the tendency to diagnose fetal asphyxia too frequently, particularly in the presence of decelerations with normal FHR variability. This has the effect of elevating the cesarean section rate unnecessarily.

263

Third, response times are rarely noted in the trials. Clearly an asphyxiated fetus needs delivery and resuscitation before damage occurs, not according to some predetermined, arbitrary "standard" time, such as "a cesarean section performed within 30 minutes." Brain damage apparently can occur in approximately 10 minutes in the case of total cessation of oxygen delivery; if our obstetric facilities cannot achieve delivery within this critical period, the fault does not rest with electronic FHR monitoring. Many of the intrapartum stillbirths in recent trials may well have been avoided with ideal response times, but such are either not discussed or are discussed in relation to a time frame that is more dependent on obstetric practicality than on biologic (i.e., fetal) need.

The "gold standard" evidence for efficacy of a medical treatment (grade 1 quality of evidence of the U.S. Preventive Services Task Force) is demonstration of efficacy in at least one well-designed randomized controlled trial. The epidemiologic planning of the FHR monitoring trials may not be able to be faulted in general, but certainly the definitions of FHR patterns, and algorithms for management, have varied widely in the different publications. For this reason plans have been made for the standardization of FHR pattern interpretation.[10, 11] Although this has been attempted numerous times before, definitions which are unambiguous, quantifiable, and computer compatible have not been agreed upon.

The point has been made by Paneth et al.,[11] epidemiologists, that the randomized controlled trials came too soon. In particular, three conditions regarding monitoring have not yet been met:

1. Reliability, with regard to interobserver agreement regarding the identity and meaning of FHR patterns.
2. Validity, that is, that specific FHR patterns are associated with the adverse neurologic outcome to be prevented.
3. A causal relationship between FHR patterns and adverse outcome.

Strength of agreement is measured by the $\kappa$ coefficient, which tests the null hypothesis that an observed agreement occurs by chance. Hence a coefficient of 0 represents complete independence of two observations, and a coefficient of 1 represents complete agreement. Intraobserver reliability in FHR pattern interpretation in four studies averaged 0.7 ("substantial agreement"),[11] and in FHR case management 0.58 ("moderate agreement").[7] Interobserver agreement for FHR pattern interpretation averaged 0.40 ("fair to moderate agreement"),[11] and for FHR case management,[7] 0.37 ("fair agreement"). Although these numbers cannot be used to quantify agreement, they are somewhat disappointingly low, and suggest a variation in both interpretation and management. But they do at least demonstrate that the clinicians are specific, and not random in their decisions. These observations make a strong case for FHR nomenclature standardization.

The validity of FHR monitoring regarding the association between FHR patterns and neurodevelopmental outcome has been examined in relatively few studies, covering about 800 patients.[11] In using criteria dating back to 1980, the pooled relative risk for developmental handicap in children having "abnormal" tracings was about 2. Despite this modest correlation, we are still faced with the fact that the majority of fetuses with "abnormal FHR patterns" as defined by these works will have a normal outcome.[9]

The third factor (i.e., a causal relationship between FHR patterns and adverse outcomes) needs confirmation to prove the point that interventions will prevent neurologic damage from occurring.

The most recent cumulative metaanalysis of the randomized controlled trials supports this concept, in that the relative risk of neonatal seizures in the electronically monitored group was 0.5, compared to the group managed by FHR auscultation[16] (Fig. 15–1). Though the link between neonatal seizures and long-term abnormal outcome could not be made, this minimizing of seizures is clearly a desirable outcome. Apart from the emotional impact of newborn seizures on the family, the cost of the medical workup and treatment of such infants is substantial. Clearly the overall cost–benefit relationship of this reduction in seizures needs to be addressed.

The weaknesses in the randomized trials of monitoring alluded to above make the significant and substantial reduction of seizures with FHR monitoring all the more optimistic, and one wonders if even stronger results may not be obvious with standardized interpretation, giving reliable and consistent management.

## B  Auscultation

The epidemiologic findings that electronic monitoring as it was practiced earlier had doubtful benefits and some risks have revised support for the use of FHR auscultation as a form of surveillance. However, there is no evidence from a randomized controlled trial that auscultation is any more effective than no auscultation, and its risks (e.g., of increasing unnecessary cesarean sections) have not been determined. In a very large survey of nearly 25,000 pregnancies over 30 years ago, Benson and coworkers[3] concluded that FHR auscultation was not effective in detecting fetal ill health except in extreme degrees of bradycardia. The dichotomous subtitles (" . . . life and death . . . ") of Kennedy's book over 150 years ago presages knowledge of the inability to make intermediate diagnoses with auscultation (Fig. 15–2).

Auscultation is proposed as an appropriate or recommended means of surveillance, particularly in the "low-risk" patient, by national organizations in both the United States and Canada. The Society of Obstetrics and

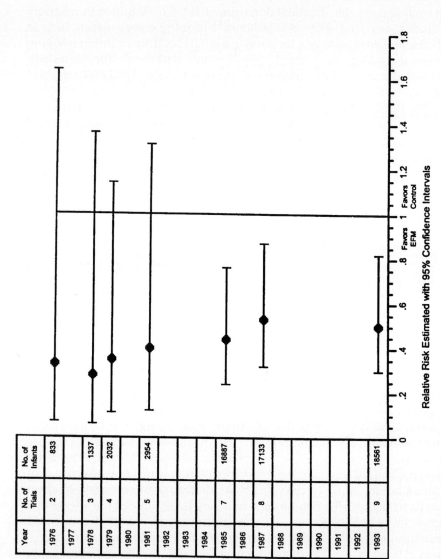

**FIGURE 15–1.** Cumulative metaanalysis of nine trials of electronic fetal monitoring (EFM) compared to FHR auscultation in the prevention of neonatal seizures. Relative risk estimated with 95% confidence intervals. (From Thacker SB, Stroup DF, Peterson HB. Efficacy and safety of intrapartum electronic fetal monitoring: An update. Obstet Gynecol 1995; 86:613–620. Reproduced by permission.)

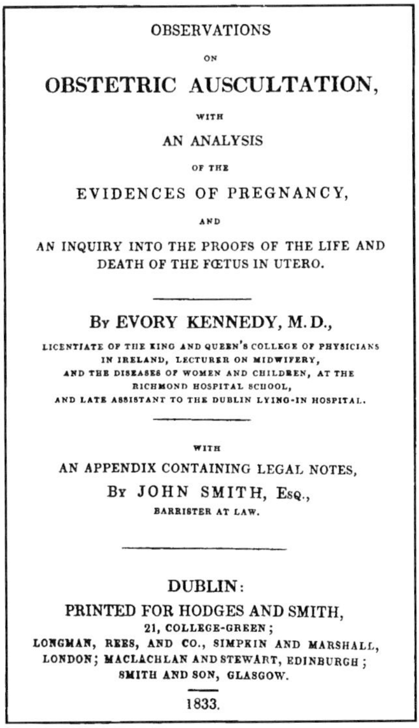

FIGURE 15–2. Title page of a text by one of the earliest proponents of the use of FHR auscultation in obstetric practice. (Figure by courtesy of Dr. L. Longo, Loma Linda University, Loma Linda, California.)

OBSERVATIONS
ON
**OBSTETRIC AUSCULTATION,**
WITH
AN ANALYSIS
OF THE
EVIDENCES OF PREGNANCY,
AND
AN INQUIRY INTO THE PROOFS OF THE LIFE AND
DEATH OF THE FŒTUS IN UTERO.

By EVORY KENNEDY, M.D.,
LICENTIATE OF THE KING AND QUEEN'S COLLEGE OF PHYSICIANS
IN IRELAND, LECTURER ON MIDWIFERY,
AND THE DISEASES OF WOMEN AND CHILDREN, AT THE
RICHMOND HOSPITAL SCHOOL,
AND LATE ASSISTANT TO THE DUBLIN LYING-IN HOSPITAL.

WITH
AN APPENDIX CONTAINING LEGAL NOTES,
By JOHN SMITH, ESQ.,
BARRISTER AT LAW.

DUBLIN:
PRINTED FOR HODGES AND SMITH,
21, COLLEGE-GREEN;
LONGMAN, REES, AND CO., SIMPKIN AND MARSHALL,
LONDON; MACLACHLAN AND STEWART, EDINBURGH;
SMITH AND SON, GLASGOW.
1833.

Gynecology of Canada report[13] believes that "intermittent auscultation is an effective technique of intrapartum fetal surveillance . . . " with specific criteria. The U.S. Preventive Services Task Force[17] states that "An auscultation schedule of every 15 minutes in the first stage of labor and every 5 minutes in the second stage has proved effective in clinical trials."

The American College of Obstetricians and Gynecologists Technical Bulletin[1] is a little less certain about the efficacy of auscultation, considering intermittent auscultation to be equivalent to electronic fetal monitoring. The most recent Technical Bulletin[2] states: "Well-controlled studies have shown that intermittent auscultation of the FHR is equivalent to continuous electronic monitoring in assessing fetal condition when performed at specific intervals with a 1:1 nurse-to-patient ratio."

These recommendations and allusions to the efficacy of auscultation are quite extraordinary in view of the fact that the technique of auscultation has not been subjected to a trial of treatment versus no auscultation, which is the appropriate trial to demonstrate efficacy. The absence of comments regarding this point are all the more extraordinary in view of the dogged insistance by monitoring opponents on the prior randomized controlled trials showing evidence of virtually no efficacy of electronic FHR monitoring. We still await a trial of electronic monitoring versus auscultation versus no FHR assessment, using rigidly defined nomenclature, modern interpretation, a rigidly followed management algorithm, and sufficient numbers. It is conceivable that such a trial may show neither electronic fetal monitoring nor auscultation is beneficial compared with no heart rate assessment at all.

---

 RISKS

## A  Cesarean Section

The major risk of electronic FHR monitoring is generally stated to be an increase in cesarean section rates, and the risk in the earliest trials was often several-fold. The relative risk in the cumulative metaanalysis of nine studies from 1976 to 1993, with over 18,000 patients, was 1.21, a gratifying decrease.[16] The relative risk of total operative deliveries was 1.23.

Another approach to determining appropriate intervention was seen in a recent study by 17 British expert obstetricians presented with 50 clinical cases.[7] The majority of experts did not recommend operative delivery in actual cases where there was a normal delivery and outcome, but did recommend operative intervention in 83 percent of cases with umbilical arterial pH <7.05. In the same study, an intelligent computer system, using FHR pattern feature extraction and a database of over 400 rules, performed at least as well as the clinicians.

## B  Infectious and Other Morbidity

Fetal morbidity has most often been sought as infectious complications through either an increased risk of chorioamnionitis, or direct fetal infection using the scalp electrode as a portal of entry. Case reports exist of herpes, group B streptococcal and gonococcal infections, and there is current concern regarding the increased risk of transmission of the human immunodeficiency virus (HIV) with the direct fetal electrode. Current recommendations are to avoid techniques resulting in breaks in the fetal skin in the presence of such infectious agents.

Maternal infectious morbidity with monitoring devices has been difficult to demonstrate because of confounding features. That is, chorioamnionitis is more common in obstructed or desultory labor, which is when internal monitoring, especially the intrauterine pressure catheter, tends to be used. However, in studies where correction has been attempted for such confounders, it is not clear whether there is an increase in maternal infection.[14] As in any aspect of medicine, the benefits of the use of monitoring in avoiding asphyxial morbidity must be weighed against any infectious morbidity.

Mechanical morbidity with the intrauterine pressure catheter is a rare but still present complication.[4] The catheter insertion has been associated with uterine perforation, placental laceration, and abruption.

## C  Intrusiveness of Fetal Heart Rate Monitoring

The use of a technological device during one of the most intimate experiences of a couple's life presents a distinct hazard of interfering with family and physician–patient interaction, and dehumanizing the birth process. For this reason the monitor must never assume the central point of labor and delivery, but should be ancillary and subservient to the couple's experience. All attendants should maintain an appropriate social interaction with the patient and make it obvious that she is more important than the machine (e.g., by making eye contact predominantly with her and not the record during examinations). Another way to minimize intrusiveness is to interpret knowledgeably, minimizing dramatic comments and activities.

 ## RECOMMENDATIONS FOR USAGE OF FETAL HEART RATE MONITORING

The almost dichotomous views of the proponents and opponents of electronic FHR monitoring can make it difficult for the practicing obstetrician to take a stand in his or her practice. Based on current recommendations physicians could opt for universal monitoring, or monitoring only high-risk patients, or not even using electronic monitoring at all. However, if they choose any of these courses, they must do so from a firm base of experience and knowledge of the literature on the subject. Few obstetricians opt for no electronic monitoring because they feel legally vulnerable. From the nursing care point of view electronic monitoring is logistically easier than intermittent auscultation.

Reasonable current recommendations are as follows:

On admission to rule out labor, or in a patient in actual labor, an FHR record with either external or internal monitoring should be documented for approximately 20 minutes. This practice has recently been termed the *admission test,* and though it is popular, there is no incontrovertible evidence of its efficacy. It is coupled sometimes with vibroacoustic stimulation.[5, 6, 12] In the case of an at-risk patient, the monitoring should continue throughout labor, although this need not be obsessively so in all cases. There are difficulties with the definition of "high risk"; suffice it to say that such a patient is one who has a condition listed in publications on the subject. Should the contractions be obvious and the FHR pattern be "normal" (normal rate, normal FHR variability, and absence of periodic changes except accelerations), the tokodynamometer need not be placed. The need for the tokodynamometer to measure contraction frequency, or for the intrauterine pressure catheter to measure intrauterine pressure, arises when labor progress is inappropriate (see Chapter 14).

For a low-risk patient who continues to be low risk in that she does not develop any abnormality of labor or have risk factors appearing subsequently, electronic FHR monitoring may be intermittent. In such cases a short recorded strip of approximately 5 minutes every 30 minutes or in accordance with the hospital's policy or American College of Obstetricians and Gynecologists recommendation[1, 2] for frequency of evaluation of FHR should be sufficient. Should equivocal changes in these short strips occur, continuous electronic FHR monitoring should be instituted until the condition of the fetus is resolved. During the second stage of labor, the frequency or recording needs to be increased in accordance with the hospital's auscultation protocol. We believe, however, that when the second stage exceeds about an hour, the institution of continuous monitoring is advisable.

As noted above, every effort should be made to minimize the intrusiveness of the monitor and associated activities, because some couples find monitoring to be at variance with their wishes for a natural birth with minimal interference.

Perhaps the most difficult aspect of monitoring is recognizing and predicting the fetus who is at risk of asphyxial damage without excessively overcalling the situation. The crucial step in this regard is in projecting the potential for asphyxia decompensation. This requires a dynamic approach to FHR interpretation, recognizing that oxygen levels in the fetus are continuously variable—from moment to moment, with contractions, and with longer cycles. Appropriate interpretation also requires an understanding of the evolution of FHR patterns in relation to progressive decreases in oxygenation, for example, in the initially normoxic fetus, the deepening of decelerations, the subsequent intermittent decrease or loss of variability, and finally the absence of variability as described above (see Chapter 11).

With careful interpretation and conservative management, we believe many of the rare cases of intrapartum asphyxia developing during labor can be recognized and, in many cases, intervention can be carried out before asphyxial damage occurs. This goal need not be achieved at the expense of excessive cesarean section rates and other potential morbidity.

# REFERENCES

**1.** American College of Obstetricians and Gynecologists. Intrapartum fetal heart rate monitoring. ACOG Technical Bulletin No. 132, 1989.

2. American College of Obstetricians and Gynecologists. Fetal heart rate patterns: Monitoring, interpretation and management. ACOG Technical Bulletin No. 207, 1995.

3. Benson RC, Shubeck F, Deutschberger J, et al. Fetal heart rate as a predictor of fetal distress. Obstet Gynecol 1968; 32:259–266.

4. Handwerker SM, Selick AM. Placental abruption after insertion of catheter tip intrauterine pressure transducers. J Reprod Med 1995; 40:845–849.

5. Ingemarsson I, Arulkumaran S, Ingemarsson E, et al. Admission test: a screening test for fetal distress in labor. Obstet Gynecol 1986; 68:801–806.

6. Ingemarsson I, Arulkumaran S, Paul RH, et al. Fetal acoustic stimulation in early labor in patients screened with the admission test. Am J Obstet Gynecol 1988; 158:70–74.

7. Keith RDF, Beckley S, Garibaldi JM, et al. A multicentre comparative study of 17 experts and an intelligent computer system for managing labour using the cardiotocogram. Br J Obstet Gynaecol 1995; 102:688–700.

8. Leveno KJ, Cunningham FG, Nelson S, et al. A prospective comparison of selective and universal electronic fetal monitoring in 34,995 pregnancies. N Engl J Med 1986; 315:615–619.

9. Lumley J. Does continuous intrapartum fetal monitoring predict long-term neurological disorders? Paed Perinat Epidemiol 1988; 2:299–307.

10. National Institutes of Health Research Planning Workshop. Electronic fetal heart rate monitoring: Research guidelines for interpretation. Am J Obstet Gynecol, in press, 1997.

11. Paneth N, Bommarito M, Stricker J. Electronic fetal monitoring and later outcome. Clin Invest Med 1993; 16:159–165.

12. Sarno AP, Ahn MO, Phelan JP, Paul RH. Fetal acoustic stimulation in the early intrapartum period as a predictor of subsequent fetal condition. Am J Obstet Gynecol 1990; 162:762–767.

13. Society of Obstetricians and Gynaecologists of Canada Policy Statement. Fetal Health Surveillance in Labour. J SOGC 1995; 17:865–901.

14. Sweet RL, Gibbs RS. Infectious Diseases of the Female Genital Tract. 3rd ed. Williams & Wilkins, Baltimore, 1995.

15. Thacker SB. The efficacy of intrapartum fetal monitoring. Am J Obstet Gynecol 1987; 156:24–30.

16. Thacker SB, Stroup DF, Peterson HB. Efficacy and safety of intrapartum electronic fetal monitoring: An update. Obstet Gynecol 1995; 86:613–620.

17. United States Preventive Services Task Force. Guide to Clinical Preventive Services. 39. Screening for fetal distress. 1989, pp. 157–160.

# ■ *Chapter Sixteen*

# Legal Aspects

Malpractice litigation is a current fact of life for obstetricians, midwives, obstetric nurses, and hospitals. The number of obstetric cases and financial settlements are among the highest for any field of medicine, primarily because of the high cost of lifetime care for an abnormal or damaged newborn. Discussion of purely legal aspects of fetal heart rate (FHR) monitoring is beyond the scope of this work, and has been covered elsewhere.[1] However, we will discuss a number of obstetrical and hospital practices which have litigational importance.

## I THE FETAL HEART RATE RECORD

The most prevalent current opinion is that the FHR record should be retained, either in its raw state or some form of copy. Copying can be done either by photographic process or on disk, both of which are conveniently available. In years past there had been some views that only a summary of the record need be kept, such as is done with the analysis of electro-cardiograms or Intensive Care Unit monitoring records, and that the raw record could be discarded. However, for various reasons this opinion has not gained much support, and both defense and plaintiff parties prefer its preservation.

There appear to be a number of reasons for this view. First, the analysis of an FHR record is dynamic, rather than static, and the provision of a comprehensive summary over many hours of labor can be quite time consuming. The summary would need to be not only descriptive, but also interpretative, which prolongs the preparation time. Some hospital forms have check boxes at specific intervals of 15 minutes, where abbreviations can be inserted, but these are usually used by the nursing staff rather than the physician. Physician charting is conventionally in handwritten or dictated notes. In the case of a discrepancy in interpretation between the nurse and physician, the only way to adjudicate the appropriateness of the differences is by reference to the original record.

A second reason for retention of the FHR record is that a number of notations are often contained on it—of blood pressure, maternal position, vaginal exam results, etc. This is a convenience in labor management and review, and we believe it should not be discouraged. Some monitors have the capacity to print items directly on the record, and most monitors now have an automatic time clock, which allows the most accurate timing of events if it is adjusted to the correct time.

A third reason to retain the record is that a discarded or lost record may be interpreted as a deliberate act to remove facts that would be detrimental to the defense. Absence of the record may make defense quite difficult, unless the written description and interpretation is comprehensive.

The clock on the monitor is an important advance, but its presence can be a detriment unless it is correctly set. This is a simple procedure, and a much more effective way of reconstructing the events during labor than hand written times. It needs to be recognized, however, that it is unusual to have all timepieces in the obstetric area synchronized, so there is frequently a few minutes discrepancy between the clocks of the monitor, the anesthesiologist, the nurse, and the delivery room wall. Timing of events may be important in reconstructing a case, particularly in cases where timely intervention is being reviewed.

## II   CHARTING

It is platitudinous to state that charting should be timely and comprehensive, but this becomes an important point in many legal reviews of cases. Nursing charting has reached a high degree of excellence, with the use of forms and check boxes to ensure timely entries.

Physician and midwife charting usually takes the form of written or dictated entries, with the dictation usually restricted to an admission note, a discharge note, an operative note, and sometimes a delivery note. Written notes, even if quite brief, can be extremely valuable in reconstructing the health care team's opinions of fetal status during labor, particularly in the presence of variant patterns (see Chapter 9).

The interpretation of the patterns should be descriptive (i.e., variable decelerations of x beats/min depth, y sec duration, and z% persistence, rather than "cord compression patterns." In addition, there should be some indication of the medical interpretation of the patterns, and, if appropriate, the trend in the pattern over time, and a plan.

One approach to the interpretation is to use terminology for diagnoses as outlined in Table 11–1. The plan could also be modified from that outlined in the "action" column in Table 11–2. These suggestions are but one approach, and others are clearly acceptable. An important principle is that notes should reflect the interpretation of the pattern, the diagnosis of the fetal state of oxygenation, and the plan of action, if it is to be altered from that preceding.

An established principle in medicine is to be relatively monosyllabic or even silent in the face of normal findings. Hence in the presence of a normal pattern (see Chapter 9), the notation "normal FHR" is sufficient, and no action or plan need necessarily be stated, as it is assumed one will allow nature to take its course, or that any current plan will continue.

## III   UMBILICAL CORD BLOOD ACID-BASE STATUS

There is now a well-established use of umbilical cord blood gases in case and management review, quality assurance and improvement, confirmation of or ruling out of asphyxia as a cause of newborn depression, research, and even intellectual curiosity regarding fetal life. Blood gases also can play a useful role in medicolegal litigation in cases where there is an allegation of mismanagement causing intrapartum asphyxia lasting until the time of birth. Normal blood gases (see Chapter 6) essentially rule out such intra-partum asphyxia, and in fact values higher than those quoted as being associated with brain damage (see Chapter 10) support the absence of asphyxia as a cause of subsequent infant neurologic morbidity. On the other hand, profound acidosis (e.g., pH <6.80, base excess < $-20$ m Eq $\cdot$ L$^{-1}$) supports a diagnosis of substantial intrapartum asphyxia at the time of birth.

Our recommendation is to obtain cord blood gases at all deliveries, if logistically and financially feasible. If such a course is not possible, then we recommend they be obtained on all depressed (low Apgar) babies, and those with an FHR pattern that suggests decompensation. Many clinicians would also recommend cord blood gases in such situations as cesarean section or operative vaginal deliveries, and in any variant patterns. If logistics or finances dictate only one specimen, then the umbilical artery is preferable, because it represents blood coming from the fetus, and there can be wide discrepancies between the values in the umbilical vein and artery under conditions of poor umbilical blood flow (see Chapter 8).

# IV THE EXPERT SYSTEM

Under the current tort system each side, plaintiff and defense, must obtain opinions from experts, and they have the right to use them in court to support their case, if they so desire. This has a great deal of appeal, in that experts can educate the judge and jury about the complexities of a case, and explain factors with which members of the court are generally unfamiliar. The adversarial system should be not unlike that which occurs in hospital case reviews, or rounds, where physicians relatively informally present their different views, and in open discussion generally reach a consensus about a case. The system should also ideally be like the discussions occurring in scientific meetings, where the acceptance of demonstrated facts is even more rigid than in medicine, because in medicine usually decisions must be made, for better or worse, on the basis of imperfect or partial data, and uncertain knowledge.

A number of factors prevent this approach toward the ideal system. The attorneys for each side can consult various experts, and only use in court those whose opinions support their case, discarding the others. Those experts discarded by one side by convention cannot be used by the other side. The usual explanation is that they may have been given privileged information by the first consultor.

A second difficulty is that an expert is anyone who the attorney can convince the court is indeed one. There is no judgment by peers about the authority of the expert, except in the most general sense in that the curriculum vitae is usually presented to the court. However, it is then up to the court to judge the authoritativeness of the expert, and this in itself can be an exceedingly difficult task.

These difficulties have given rise to the concept and presence of "hired guns," who will say things in court which would be sufficient to have them laughed out of hospital rounds, or become the pariahs of a scientific meeting. They tend to specialize in testifying for only one side, either defense or plaintiff. There have been discussions about how to identify and police such people,[2] but so far no system has been devised to judge the expertise of the experts, and ensure their knowledge of current medical opinion.

From the point of view of FHR monitoring, several things may help this situation. First, the standardization of FHR pattern nomenclature (see Chapter 9) will ensure we are all talking the same language. Second, the use of intelligent computer systems, with algorithms devised by experts and validated in appropriate trials, should help to standardize management[3] and reduce the current dichotomous opinions of experts.

Until then, all we can do is develop a Panglossian attitude, treat our patients with great respect, give full and informed consent, learn the latest about FHR monitoring, manage cases to the best of our ability and knowledge, and write good brief notes.

## REFERENCES

1. Fineberg KS, Peters JD, Wellson JR, Kroll DA. Obstetrics/Gynecology and the Law. Health Administration Press. Ann Arbor, Michigan 1984, p. 616.

2. Fisher CW, Dombrowski MP, Jaszczak SE, et al. The expert witness: Real issues and suggestions. Am J Obstet Gynecol 1995; 172:792–800.

3. Keith RDF, Beckley S, Garibaldi JM, et al. A multicentre comparative study of 17 experts and an intelligent computer system for managing labor using the cardiotocogram. Br J Obstet Gynaecol 1995; 102:688–700.

# ■ Index